The Third Reich

IN THE UNCONSCIOUS

The Third Reich in the Unconscious

TRANSGENERATIONAL TRANSMISSION AND ITS CONSEQUENCES

VAMIK D. VOLKAN, GABRIELE AST, AND WILLIAM F. GREER, JR.

Routledge
Taylor & Francis Group
NEW YORK AND LONDON

Published in 2002 by Brunner-Routledge

This edition published 2011 by Routledge:

Routledge
Taylor & Francis Group
711 Third Avenue
New York, NY 10017

Routledge
Taylor & Francis Group
27 Church Road
Hove, East Sussex BN3 2FA

First issued in paperback 2014

Routledge is an imprint of the Taylor and Francis Group, an informa business

Library of Congress Cataloging-in-Publication Data

Volkan, Vamık D., 1932–
The Third Reich in the unconscious : transgenerational transmission and its consequences / Vamık D. Volkan, Gabriele Ast, and William F. Greer, Jr.
p. cm.
Includes bibliographical references and indexes.
ISBN 1-58391-334-3
1. Social psychiatry—Germany—Case studies. 2. Psychoanalysis—Case studies. 3. National socialism—Psychological aspects. 4. World War, 1939–1945—Germany—Psychological aspects. 5. Psychotherapy patients—Family relationships. 6. Intergenerational relations. I. Ast, Gabriele. II. Greer, William F. III. Title.

RC455 .V654 2002
616.89′00943—dc21

2001052501

ISBN 13: 978-1-583-91334-5 (hbk)
ISBN 13: 978-0-415-76350-9 (pbk)

Contents

About the Authors

Vamık D. Volkan, M.D., is professor of psychiatry at the University of Virginia and director of the Center for the Study of Mind and Human Interaction (CSMHI), University of Virginia School of Medicine, Charlottesville, Virginia. He is a training and supervising analyst at the Washington Psychoanalytic Institute and a former president of both the International Society of Political Psychology (ISPP) and the Virginia Psychoanalytic Society. Dr. Volkan is the recipient of many awards, including the ISPP's Nevitt Sanford Award for his work on political psychology (1994), the American Orthopsychiatric Association's Max Hayman Award for outstanding contribution to the psychology of racism and genocide (1995), the American Anthropological Association's L. Bryce Boyer Award for his study of post-Ceaușescu Romania (1996), and the Margaret Mahler Literature Prize (1999) for his writings on clinical issues. In 2000, he served as an Inaugural Yitzhak Rabin Fellow at the Rabin Center in Israel. He is the author or coauthor of 24 books and the editor or coeditor of 7 more.

Gabriele Ast, M.D., is a psychoanalyst and family practice physician in private practice in Münich, Germany. Formerly, she was a faculty member of the Department of Psychotherapy and Psychosomatics at the Psychiatric Hospital, Ludwig Maximilian University, Münich. She has coauthored three books: one on borderline personality organization, one on narcissistic conditions, and one on sibling relationships.

William F. Greer, Jr., Ph.D., is assistant professor, Community Faculty, at the Medical College of Hampton Roads, Norfolk, Virginia. A clinical associate member of the Virginia Psychoanalytic Society, he also maintains a private practice in Hampton, Virginia.

Acknowledgments

FOR MORE THAN 25 YEARS, senior author Vamık Volkan has studied the relationships between individual and large-group (e.g., ethnic or national group) psychology, as well as between societies and individuals massively traumatized by war or warlike situations. In 1990, he and Gabriele Ast initiated a project to study the intrapsychic ramifications of the reunification of Germany. Their initial findings suggested that among the Germans they interviewed, reunification had stimulated the appearance of many images of and feelings about the Third Reich. It seemed as if West Germans had placed the blame for the Nazi period on East Germans, and vice versa; each side had, in general, denied its own involvement in and culpability for the Nazi past, and reunification seemed to threaten these denials. Intervening circumstances prevented Volkan and Ast's project from being completed; during their work, however, they became aware of a significant "silence" blanketing Third Reich–related images in Germany. It was this uncompleted work that eventually led to the present project.

Vamık Volkan and Gabriele Ast have previously coauthored three books. They are joined in this book's examination of an important, but relatively ignored, area of interdependence between individual and large-group psychologies by William Greer, who has worked closely with Dr. Volkan for 15 years.

The authors are grateful to Sabine X., a psychoanalytic colleague, for giving permission to tell her story. They also thank the core members of Psychotherapeutischer Arbeitskreis für Betroffene des Holocaust (PAKH) (Psychotherapeutic Study Group for People Affected by the Holocaust)—Bernd Klose, Liliane Opher-Cohn, Johannes Pfäfflin, Peter Pogány-Wnendt, and Bernd Sonntag—who gave permission to report their experience of organizing a symposium to address German "speechlessness" on the subject of the Nazi regime and the Holocaust.

The authors would also like to thank Bruce Edwards and Joy Boissevain, former and current managing editors of the journal *Mind and Human Interaction*, respectively, as well as Susan Stine, administrative assistant to Dr. Volkan at the Center for the Study of Mind and Human Interaction at the University of Virginia, all of whom have demonstrated their customary diligence in working on this manuscript. Danielle Pelfrey Duryea of the University of Virginia Department of English helped us greatly by being responsible for the final editing of this book; we are grateful to her, and to Shelley Staples, who also assisted us in the final editing process.

Foreword

IRA BRENNER, M.D.

Clinical Associate Professor of Psychiatry
Jefferson Medical College, Philadelphia, Pennsylvania

Executive Director
Training and Supervising Analyst
Philadelphia Psychoanalytic Institute

IT IS AN HONOR TO WRITE THIS FOREWORD, not only because of the significance of this topic to me personally and professionally, but also because of the nature of my relationship with Vamık Volkan, the senior coauthor. His work on pathological mourning, his theoretical contributions to object relations theory, and his application of this deep understanding of the psyche to the problems of ethnic identity, ethnic conflict, and large-group processes need no introduction; his international reputation has been well established for many years and a number of his contributions have already become classics. I have known him personally for about 25 years—since I was a resident in psychiatry, when his brilliance, like a beacon, first illuminated the path of my career. He helped me recognize some of my own potential and pointed me in the direction of becoming a psychoanalyst. After leaving his formal tutelage, I pursued the study of psychic trauma, and so I feel very gratified as well to see some of my own contributions to the study of the Holocaust, or the *Shoah*, cited in this volume.

Students of Adolf Hitler's life have noted that he had an uncanny ability to ignite large crowds and perhaps an even greater ability to sense the potential for moral corruptibility and decay in individuals when he met with them one-on-one. He was described as hypnotic, irresistible, and much more intelligent than is often acknowledged now. And if it is true that the character of the leader is reflected in his policies, laws, and governance, then one may see the amplification of his psyche during the "black and red plague" that spread through Europe between 1933 and 1945. Warding off the devastating effect of malignant humiliation stemming from his childhood, Hitler's dream of the Aryan superrace "justified" the subjugation, humiliation, and liquidation of others, others deemed inferior and "unworthy of life": Jews, Gypsies, homosexuals, the handicapped, and the mentally ill. The extent to which the dominant group could be induced and seduced into committing atrocities against other human beings reached unprecedented heights during the Third Reich. The darkest side of human nature was brought forth in bold relief by the leaders of this regime: a confirmation of that most awesome, murderous potential that resides in our species. It is as though Hitler himself had offered this interpretation to us about the human race; yet there was—and, amazingly, still is—enormous resistance to accepting it. Now, almost 60 years after the last crematoria in Auschwitz has cooled, and despite the fact that the memories of the witnesses are dimming, there is no lack of interest in these most haunting moments of the twentieth century. On the contrary, contemporary reports of genocidal persecution are an ever-growing ripple left by the Führer on the surface of modern civilization. The Holocaust is a constant reminder of this basic fact about the human animal, and perhaps it is because this fact is as fundamental as the cosmic battle between Eros and Thanatos that it has become so deeply rooted in the mind.

The symbols and images of the Third Reich, assisted by the modern media, have become almost universally etched into the global consciousness. The ways in which those who have been directly affected incorporate this material and unconsciously transmit it to succeeding generations form a central part of this book, but the ways in which those with no connection with the Third Reich also incorporate those images are under examination here, too. Sandwiched between rich theoretical and technical discussions, the detailed clinical case material includes children of Jewish survivors, a Jewish child survivor, and a very rare psychoanalytic study of a German "Gypsy" who was successfully treated by Dr. Ast. The often overlooked groups of Gypsy peoples even have a specific name for their genocidal persecution—*Porraimos*, "the devouring"—but in the absence of the written tradition of the Jews, their trauma has not been recorded as thoroughly. This book is, therefore, an important addition to the growing literature that documents their suffering as well. The self-analysis of a German woman psychoanalyst is yet another unusual contribution to a more well-known area, highlighting the different challenges that the offspring of ethnic Germans who lived through the Third Reich have, compared to children of survivors. The latter deal with the essentially irrational nature of their parents' survivor guilt, whereas the former have to reconcile themselves to the great possibility of their parents' moral degradation, a different superego problem.

My own work in this area started with the Group for the Psychoanalytic Study of the Effects of the Holocaust on the Second Generation, co-chaired by Judith Kestenberg, Martin Bergmann, and Milton Jucovy. We endeavored to tease out "private pathology" from "Holocaust pathology," which was ascribed to a phenomenon coined by Kestenberg as the "transposition." In this model, the survivor parents were seen as transmitting their trauma unconsciously to the developing child, who grew up living both in the present and in the parents' traumatic Holocaust past. These children might enter a psychological time tunnel, as it were, and weave their parents' past into their own developmental experience, as well as unconsciously relive elements of the parents' survival experience during corresponding milestones in their own lives. For example, when the child reached the age of the parent when the parent's traumatic events—for example, deportation, incarceration in a concentration camp, specific life-threatening shock trauma, witnessing the death of loved ones—occurred, the child might develop symptoms or enact situations that brought on dire consequences. One such patient of mine repeatedly provoked and narrowly escaped entanglements with the law and was eventually jailed at the very age his father had been during his hiding, escape, and subsequent capture by the Gestapo. As a result, I felt it to be imperative to help the analyzand reconstruct in great detail his parent's Holocaust experience, as well as his own childhood fantasy life. A number of very talented "outsider" analysts who presented their own case material to the group regularly challenged this unique feature of analyses of the second generation, arguing that since analysis deals with the realm of psychic reality only, we were introducing an unnecessary element that only "muddied the waters" and was unnecessary for successful treatment. As persuasive as many of these arguments were, we nevertheless felt that much would have remained unanalyzed without this extra step, which required an understanding of historical reality.

Volkan and his associates confront this question from another angle, which has broad technical implications. By introducing their new theory "that images of the Nazi period transmitted from generation to generation in large groups affected by the Third Reich initiate—and, indeed, actually become—*unconscious fantasies,*" they maintain that such fantasies, "developed solely by the offspring, reflect the general history of the large group to which [the child] belongs; their sources are not limited to direct ancestors' actual personal experiences" (p. 23). Volkan's seminal contribution of the "chosen trauma," described in chapter 4, elaborates upon this concept. This perspective, I believe, is a compromise position that necessitates the analyst's thorough understanding and appreciation of the shared historical facts involved, but perhaps does not demand as thorough an examination of the parents' specific history. By focusing on general themes and the integration of perpetrator and victim self-representations, such an approach can be applied broadly to those not directly affected by the Holocaust as well. The reader will see this principle in operation in the clinical material, and it is especially well elucidated in Dr. Greer's outstanding analytic work with "Leo," recounted in chapter 6.

Chapter 5's case history of Jacob, who lived in hiding with his parents for about the first 18 months of his life, raises important questions about children of survivors versus child survivors. The former were born after the war but often grew up with an uncanny sense of having "been there" and having a wish to rescue their parents; the latter were born during the war but may have grown up in denial of having been there or minimizing any role in their own survival, since many were told they were too young to remember and "should not" have been affected in any way. Early studies of members of the former group led researchers to make dire predictions about their future mental health, which have not been borne out; the latter group was virtually overlooked by the early researchers and became an invisible remnant whose experience was not validated. The formation of specific organizations and support groups for child survivors also lagged behind comparable structures for adult survivors and the second generation. Jacob would by definition have been an infant survivor; he grew up with second-hand memories of his parents' memories and had only somatic memories of his own experience, which came out in dreams and in the transference. He had slept in a dresser drawer and, as a crying infant, was almost choked to death by his father in order to avoid detection by the Gestapo. He suffered primarily from his own early life-threatening trauma, but also from the transmission from his parents, as would typically be seen in the second generation also. This "double dose," as it were, complicated his development and made it impossible for him to mourn the untimely death of his father. Although this reveals important history about his parents and his harrowing young life, certain details are not available that might have lent more understanding to the dynamics and timing of his suicide attempt at age 27 and his abandonment of treatment. Although it is admittedly speculative, but based on the unconscious repetition psychoanalysts have seen in such cases, I would wonder if Jacob's father was also about age 27 when, while in hiding, he felt he had to strangle Jacob to save the family. If Jacob's overdose had been successful, he would have stopped breathing again; he would have completed the self-contained enactment of the father having to sacrifice his son. It is also not known how much his wife wanted a child, how afraid the recently married Jacob was that he, too, might have to kill his own child, and to what extent he symbolically sacrificed himself to prevent a recurrence. Furthermore, did the length of time in treatment—before he "escaped" and went back into hiding once again in order to avoid the intolerable affects associated with his memories—correspond to the length of time he was in hiding as an infant? And if so, could bringing this fact to his attention possibly have helped him suppress his urge to run away? Teasing out the disguised patterns of symbolic reliving of trauma may reveal the blueprint of a personal and an intergenerational repetition compulsion that could be an invaluable clinical guide.

Chapter 9 of this book chronicles the planning of an unusual conference in Germany during the summer of 1998 by a group of children of Holocaust survivors and children of ethnic Germans who lived through World War II. Their struggles over coming together, finding a way to speak to each other, and planning the conference, a microcosm of the issues at hand, were carefully supervised by Dr. Volkan. On a personal note, I wish to recount some of my own experiences immediately surrounding that gathering. Naturally, my awareness of the shadows of the past had become rather heightened in anticipation of this conference. During a cruise I took along the Rhine with my wife before the conference, the overwhelming majority of passengers were Germans over the age of 60, with only four of us Americans aboard this pride of the German riverboat fleet. In keeping with a bit of an ethnic stereotype, the accommodations were rather spartan but meticulously clean. The food was outstanding, the service was impeccable, and we were on schedule for every stop along the way; the operation ran like clockwork. There was unlimited beer and wine with every meal, and everyone was very jovial. The weather was superb, and we spent glorious days lounging on the deck by the pool watching the castles go by. It was idyllic. When we docked, our tour guides were extremely knowledgeable and went into great detail about the historical significance of each church, castle, or monument we saw, except that they had virtually nothing to say about what had been destroyed as a result of the war. If a passing comment such as "And this was built after 1945 . . . " was made, it was said so quickly that the guide was on to the next topic before one had time to react or inquire further. To have been too curious about their omissions, it felt to me, would have been to "rock the boat" and to spoil the jolly mood that prevailed.

One night we were docked at a small town near the French border, and our evening's entertainment was a local group of Alsatian dancers dressed in distinctive native garb. This troupe of dark-haired "foreigners" failed to keep the attention of a large segment of the inebriated audience, the members of which became restless and progressively louder in the nightclub. It was the first overt sign of rudeness, disrespect, or intolerance we had seen. During the dancers' last number prior to intermission, one of the oldest men in the audience broke out into what sounded like a popular beer-drinking song. Almost as though on cue, he was immediately joined by members of the crowd, who locked arms and drowned out the other music. At this point, my own images of the Third Reich were activated; I got an eerie feeling and suddenly felt surrounded, in hostile territory. I imagined that I was in the middle of a Hitler rally, like the one attended by Leo's father. I felt a sudden urge to leave the ship. Of course, it was rather late, but it became imperative to me to find some evidence of Jewish life in this very old town, dominated by a huge medieval cathedral. At that moment, in my regression, I wondered if there were any traces of Jews left in Germany or whether it truly had become *Judenrein* ("free of Jews"). Curiously, we noted on the map that here in Speyer was the excavation of an eleventh-century ritual bath, or *mikveh*, which was the oldest evidence of Jewish life in the Rhine River valley. Armed with flashlights and wandering through the empty cobblestone streets at midnight on this silent, steamy summer night, I realized that my mission to find the *Judenstrasse* ("Jewish Street") felt like an antidote to the nationalistic fervor of the Germans that I had read into the scene at the nightclub. When we finally reached the Jewish landmark, I was dismayed to see that the "entrance" was a makeshift plywood door secured with a padlock, with handwritten information scrawled on it with a marking pen. It looked pathetic compared to the grandeur of the architecture devoted to Christianity and seemed more like a boarded-up building defaced with anti-Semitic graffiti after a night of looting and vandalism. In my mind, an image of *Kristallnacht*, the national pogrom in Germany on November 9, 1938, became superimposed on this humble archaeological vestige of my wandering ancestors.

Strangely reassured nonetheless—because *something* indeed had survived—I felt quietly triumphant and returned to the vessel fortified by this clandestine encounter with my defiant heritage. The next day, however, my reverie continued; while waiting in line for the showers before entering the pool on this scorching day, listening to everyone speaking German around me, I felt a chill as a fleeting image of prisoners calmly waiting in line to enter gas chambers disguised as showers swept through my consciousness. During our stop in Strasbourg, France, we sought out the synagogue, which was a rebuilt and impressive postwar building: concrete evidence of the renaissance of Jewish life. We were eager to tour the inside just as we had made our way through the magnificent Christian sacred places. Unfortunately, we were blocked at the door by a young man nervously smoking a cigarette behind a bullet-proof Plexiglas window, who informed us that the synagogue was closed for the summer (!). The ever-present threat of terrorism resulted in such measures; the underlying fear of being a Jew in visible public places saddened me. Nevertheless, I was heartened to see that the protective measures taken had revised the Holocaust image of the defenseless, helpless Jew in the ghetto or concentration camp.

On the long train ride back to Cologne after the cruise, I sat across from a man in his 30s who did not speak English. I tried to make conversation in my broken German, and he seemed rather friendly, pointing out the various landmarks whizzing by our windows. After several hours, I took a chance and told him I was on my way to a special conference; I showed him a copy of the conference flyer, and it was as if it caught fire in his hands. He seemed shocked by what he read and could not wait to give it back to me. He said nothing more for the rest of the trip. I felt as though I had spoiled our limited rapport by broaching the silence of the Holocaust.

While at the conference, I was discouraged from wearing my nametag in public places for fear of reprisals by anyone who might have objected to the theme of the conference or who might have made trouble for me. My nametag felt like it had become the obligatory yellow star identifying me as a Jew in Nazi-occupied Europe. The potential danger of being recognized and harassed felt very real to my German colleagues, so I quietly conformed and "went into hiding" as I walked the streets. The conference was a very successful and profoundly moving event, culminating on Saturday evening after the Sabbath with a gala dinner dance for all of the attendees. The climax of the evening was the traditional Jewish circle dance, the horah, in which children of survivors and children of Nazis literally joined hands to celebrate life. Ultimately, I left Germany this time with this hopeful image of what the future could be, and it neutralized my images of what had been during the Third Reich.

This extraordinary meeting of the second generation from both sides of the "barbed wire" would not have occurred without Vamık Volkan. Similarly, this book is also a collaborative effort of dedicated professionals who have been brought together and inspired by Dr. Volkan. It is fitting that a man of Vamık Volkan's stature would assemble two very capable coauthors to confront the legacy of Adolf Hitler. Like scientists shifting magnification on their microscopes, Drs. Volkan, Ast, and Greer offer us an examination of the intergenerational effects of the Third Reich from the large ethnic group perspective, through the small-group process, down to the tiny intrapsychic units of self- and object-representations. Drs. Volkan, Ast, and Greer have created and filled a very important niche in the literature regarding the long-term effects of this type of trauma; their blueprint will guide members of all disciplines who want to understand and help those throughout the world who have been affected by man-made large-group catastrophes. This volume bears Dr. Volkan's unique imprimatur and is destined to become another invaluable contribution to the human sciences.

Introduction

As IS WELL-KNOWN, the Allies' defeat of the Third Reich in 1945 brought an end not only to World War II, but also to what we now know as the Holocaust: the unprecedented, systematic attempt to achieve "racial purity" through the extermination of millions of innocent people. Under the Third Reich descent alone would condemn a person to certain death. Reduced, in the eyes of their persecutors, to the lowest form of life, entire peoples—as well as homosexuals and those with physical and mental anomalies—were thought of as a threat to the "Aryan race"; as invaders of the "Aryan body," they were to be totally and completely annihilated in order to purge the German genetic pool of their supposed taint. Thus the Nazis' so-called Final Solution represented an utter and total debasement and dehumanization of certain groups of people by another group: a cataclysmic event that has changed the shape of human history forever (Moses, 1993).

For psychoanalysts and other mental health workers, the survivors of Nazi concentration camps generated a hitherto unprecedented need to study individual and mass reaction to overwhelming stress brought about by politically motivated human cruelty. Persecution in its various forms—the relentless pursuit of people in hiding, the erosion of emotional health and intellectual strength, mass expulsion, and economic assault—all demanded to be studied in psychodynamic terms. Yet it should not come entirely as a surprise that when Jews and other members of persecuted groups were rescued from the concentration camps, no one seriously considered the psychological plight of these victims, for their physical trauma was so terribly visible. Far less obvious, but no less real, was the massive psychological trauma that they had suffered.

Psychological trauma occurs when a stimulus—one that is sudden and disruptive, one that repeats and accumulates, or both of these—arises either from an external situation or from massive inner libidinal or aggressive excitement; it overwhelms the ego's capacity to mediate between the various forces making demands upon it, creating a state of helplessness. Otto Fenichel's 1945 remarks on trauma still hold true: It is "a relative concept; factors of mental economy, dependent on constitution as well as on previous experiences and on the actual conditions before and during trauma" (p. 117), determine what degree of excitation will overtake an individual's capacity to deal with the single overwhelming event or cumulative injurious events—or injurious events that are both single and cumulative.

We speak of *massive psychic trauma* when the traumatic experience takes precedence over the individual's past predispositions, which are obliterated. Initially, the massive psychic trauma may produce similar psychological disturbances in everyone who suffers from it. Whatever ego strengths and good object relations may have existed before the experience play little or no part in determining outcome; "The regenerative powers of the ego are not limitless, the human spirit can be broken beyond repair" (Rappaport, 1968, p. 730). Even though expressions may vary in the long run, the effects of massive trauma on the directly traumatized individual do not altogether disappear with time. As Leo Rangell (1976) writes,

> In spite of the vastness of the unconscious, psychic space is limited. There is room and time in any individual for only a limited amount of cognitive ideation and a finite number of memories, fantasies, and accompanying affects. . . . Traumatic memories of any kind encroach on this psychic time-space and reduce its available quantity; this is why psychic traumata age people. (p. 315)

When people experience a massive trauma, its psychological impact takes several forms. First, many will suffer various types of post-traumatic stress disorder (PTSD), a subject studied extensively in the psychiatric and psychological literature (see Thomson, 2000, for a comprehensive review of post-traumatic symptoms). To review briefly: For those suffering from PTSD, trauma-inducing experiences resist encapsulation in the normal memory. Instead, the sufferer experiences states of hyper-arousal as the traumatic experiences resurface vividly, often unexpectedly: "It is as if the central nervous system has been reconditioned and there is no longer a baseline state of calm and comfort" (Thomson, 2000, p. 163). The regulation of emotions, consciousness, self-perception, perception of the trauma's perpetrator, relations with others, and the meaning of events all are altered.

Second, new social processes and shared behaviors may appear throughout the affected community or communities, initiated by changes in the common psychological states of the affected individuals. If what Kai Erikson (1975) called the "tissue" of the community is not broken, however, the society eventually recovers in what Williams and Parks (1975) refer to as a process of "biosocial regeneration" (p. 304). In the five years following the deaths of 116 children and 28 adults in an avalanche of coal slurry in the Welsh village of Aberfan, for example, there was a significant increase in the birthrate among women who had not themselves lost a child. Such a response to disaster is possible even when another group has inflicted the trauma intentionally. Cypriot Turks experienced a somewhat indirect biosocial regeneration during the six-year period (1963–1968) in which they were forced by Cypriot Greeks to live in isolated enclaves under subhuman conditions. Though the Cypriot Turks were massively traumatized, their "backbone" remained unbroken because of the hope that Turkey would come to their aid. Instead of bearing increased numbers of children like the inhabitants of Aberfan, they raised hundreds and hundreds of parakeets in cages—representing their "imprisoned" selves. As long as the birds (which are not native to Cyprus) sang and reproduced, Cypriot Turks' anxiety remained in check (Volkan, 1979). The impact of some disasters—both accidental man-made and intentional—may be much deeper, however. After the 1986 nuclear accident at Chernobyl—which was responsible for at least 8,000 deaths—justifiable anxiety about radiation contamination exercised a considerable influence on the social fabric of communities in and around Chernobyl. Thousands of people in neighboring Belarus, for instance, considered themselves contaminated with radiation and expressed unwillingness to have children, fearing birth defects. Thus the prior norms for finding a mate, marrying, and planning a family were significantly disrupted, and those who did have children often remained continually anxious that something "bad" would appear in their children's health. Here, instead of an adaptive biosocial regeneration, affected communities responded to trauma with what might be termed a "biosocial degeneration."

Third and finally, traumatized persons may, mostly unconsciously, oblige their descendants to resolve the directly traumatized generation's unfinished psychological tasks relating to the shared trauma—reversing helplessness, for example, or mourning various losses. Images connected with the shared trauma then become involved in what is called *transgenerational transmission*. *The Third Reich in the Unconscious* is concerned with this third expression of the psychological impact of massive trauma.

Aims and Organization of This Book

Part 1 of this book outlines the mechanics of transgenerational transmission necessary to understand the Third Reich–related case studies reported in part 2 and the therapeutic considerations discussed in part 3. In part 1, we illustrate the various types of transgenerational transmission we have observed in clinical work and review their theoretical implications. Descendants of massive trauma survivors certainly identify with their parents' (or more distant ancestors') ways of adapting to their personal traumas. But the concept of *identification* alone does not explain all the psychological processes observed in trauma survivors' offspring. Identification alone cannot explain, for example, how descendants' developmental issues related to internalized object relations, separation-individuation and psychosexual conflicts, ego or superego difficulties, early object loss, early childhood abuse, and other psychologically important traumas defensively and adaptively become condensed with the mental representations of their *large group*'s shared past history. (In the psychological literature, "large group" usually designates a gathering of 50 to 100 individuals assembled for a collective therapeutic experience; in this book, however, the term *large group* refers to any aggregate of hundreds of thousands or millions of people forming a cultural or political unity or both—e.g., an ethnic, national, or religious group.)

In part 1, we present the new theory that images of the Nazi period transmitted from generation to generation in large groups affected by the Third Reich thus initiate—and, indeed, actually become—*unconscious fantasies* (see also Auerhahn and Laub, 1998; Kogan, 2000). People into whom the mental representation of a shared traumatic event has been passed may live simultaneously in two worlds, their own and that inhabited by their ancestors (Eckstaedt, 1989; Kogan, 2000)—the former more consciously and the latter mostly unconsciously (although some individuals may also inhabit the latter consciously). They are, unbeknownst to themselves and most others, caught up in a sort of time warp involving past traumatic events visited upon the large group to which they belong, but which they themselves never directly experienced—events the "memories" of which have become literally unrememberable yet truly unforgettable. They are haunted (Abraham, 1988), as it were, by a previous generation's ghostly, traumatized aspects, which live on in their internal worlds. Maurice Apprey (1993a) observes this phenomenon in African Americans whose ancestors were victims of slavery. These unconscious fantasies, developed solely by the offspring, reflect the general history of the large group to which individuals belong; the sources of these fantasies are not limited to direct ancestors' actual personal experiences.

When such a person "lives" in the past, he or she adopts various roles—victim or victimizer, for example—and recreates mental representations of the past history in seemingly endless and various "replays" in interpersonal relations, as well as in both transference and extra-transference repetitions in treatment. In part 2 of this book, we provide detailed case histories of individuals "living in the past"; except for one, who was eight months old when World War II ended, none of these individuals—a Jenish (German "Gypsy") woman, a German woman, and three Jewish persons—lived under the Nazi regime. The report of the total analytic process in two cases and details of others serve to illustrate the intertwining of the patients' history-related unconscious fantasies with their more typical ones—personal developmental conflicts, identification with parents, and the like. Part 2's study of a group of German colleagues illustrates the degree to which the influence of the Third Reich "lives," even among those who were trained to examine their own internal worlds before becoming therapists for others.

Part 2 reports, as well, on Third Reich–related issues in four individuals whose ancestors were not directly affected by the Nazi regime. Two of these people had siblings with physical disabilities, and one of them was himself disabled, but the fourth was not Jewish, Gypsy, German, homosexual, disabled, or mentally ill—all identities or conditions that might be expected to suggest associations with the Nazis, their victims, or both. Nevertheless, all four invoked images of the Third Reich to express perceptions of psychologically "murderous" childhood environments or to relive such early relationships in their transference neuroses. To us, such cases reflect the dramatic extent to which Third Reich symbols have become generalized, even in the unconscious of individuals who neither lived under Nazi rule nor were otherwise directly affected by the Third Reich in any way.

Part 3 turns to the premises and procedures relevant for treating unconscious "carriers" of Third Reich images. We type these patients into various treatment categories and return to the cases detailed in part 2 in order to reexamine the therapeutic theory and technique applied in those courses of treatment.

The questions that have preoccupied us throughout all three sections of this study include:

- How does shared historical trauma become entwined with transgenerational transmission?
- How do individuals' own personal object relations, psychosexual or aggressive conflicts, and other developmental issues become condensed with the mental images of history that are passed to them by parents or other significant caregivers?
- When do such historical images initiate unconscious fantasies that become the dominant force determining the nature of our patients' expressions of object relations and symptoms?
- Why do some offspring adjust well to the mental images of history passed on to them, whereas others evolve psychopathologies?
- How does the existence of images of a past shared trauma among members of a large group increase individuals' investment in their large-group identity?
- How do the images of ancestors' shared trauma appear in patients' transference neuroses?
- How do attempts to modify or to work through conflicts associated with images of shared historical trauma create strong resistances to psychoanalysis or psychotherapy?
- Are there specific obstacles to the treatment of individuals whose parents or grandparents were traumatized during the Third Reich?
- What are the typical countertransference issues during the treatment of these patients?

- What is the "therapeutic play" that is necessary to treat individuals severely affected by history-related unconscious fantasies?
- Are we ready to develop strategies to tame or even to prevent pathological transgenerational transmissions of trauma?

We propose, finally, that what we have learned from investigating transgenerational transmission of Nazi-era images can be usefully extrapolated to the study of all large groups for which shared historical images have initiated unconscious fantasies and thus influence individual members' psychopathology, adaptations, or both—but *not* because other large-group historical traumas are in any way comparably catastrophic. Indeed, on the contrary, it is because of the Holocaust's very enormity that Third Reich image transmissions magnify the observable derivatives of what we understand to be a generic mechanism of transgenerational transmission. We hope to draw new attention to the significant influences of history-related unconscious conflicts on individual lives, and we believe that as a result of our contribution, psychoanalysts and psychotherapists can become more alert to the possible influence of shared historical trauma on their patients' object relations, symptoms, and character formations.

We do hope that the psychoanalysts and psychotherapists among our readers will find this volume useful in their everyday clinical work. We feel very strongly, however, that the topics we address have implications far beyond the clinician's office. Thus we have sought to make the book less technically cumbersome, in the hope that it will cast light across the disciplines on matters of societal identity and on the political and historical issues that typically follow shared massive trauma resulting from human aggression, as well as on new concepts of "preventive medicine" that can be provided to societies so traumatized. It is time—indeed, we believe it past time—for professionals in fields from mental health to diplomacy to attend to post-trauma psychological issues beyond PTSD.

Part 1

ON THE MENTAL REPRESENTATION OF HISTORY

1

Beyond PTSD

FROM TRAUMA TO TRANSGENERATIONAL TRANSMISSION

A comparison of Armenians directly affected by the 1988 earthquake with Armenians personally traumatized as a result of the Armenian–Azerbaijan ethnic conflict during the same year (Goenjian et al., 2000) concludes that, after 18 months and again after 54 months, there were no significant differences in individual "PTSD severity, profile, or course . . . between subjects exposed to severe earthquake trauma versus those exposed to severe violence" (p. 911). Such statistical studies measuring observable manifestations of trauma's lasting effects (anxiety, depression, or other signs of PTSD) are misleading, however, insofar as they do not reveal much about individual minds or hidden psychological processes; apparent symptomatic uniformity can hide significant qualitative differences. Furthermore, such studies do not illuminate the societal processes that may result from shared trauma and their long-term (transgenerational) effects. For instance, the fact that many Armenians injured in the earthquake refused to accept blood donated by Azerbaijanis suggests that the tragedy had actually enhanced ethnic feeling, including resistance to "mixing blood" with the enemy. In fact, there are various types of shared catastrophe, and they provoke various characteristic responses.

When people suffer as a result of natural disasters such as tropical storms, floods, volcanic eruptions, forest fires, and earthquakes, survivors ultimately tend to accept the event as part of their fate or as the will of God (Lifton and Olson, 1976). Even after man-made accidental disasters, such as the Chernobyl accident, survivors may blame a small number of individuals or governmental organizations for their carelessness, but fundamentally there are no "others" who have deliberately sought to hurt the victims. Though natural and accidental disasters may cause collective grief, anxiety, and change, as well as massive environmental destruction, they should, generally speaking, be differentiated from those in which the shared catastrophe results from large-group conflicts.

It is true that it can sometimes be difficult to categorize a given disaster definitively as only one type. For example, the massive August 1999 earthquake in Turkey that killed an estimated 20,000 people was, of course, a natural disaster. But it also provides an example of a man-made accidental catastrophe: Many of the buildings that collapsed during the earthquake had not been constructed according to appropriate quality standards, and it was revealed after the quake that some builders had bribed certain local authorities in order to put up these cheaper, unsafe structures.

Interestingly, the Turkish quake also stimulated changes in what had been enduring ethnic sentiments among Greeks and Turks. After the earthquake, rescue workers from around the world rushed to Turkey to help—among them, many Greeks. By publishing the pictures and stories of individual Greek rescue workers, Turkish newspapers helped to "humanize" Greeks as a group, who for decades were perceived as an enemy. Only a few years before the quake, Turkey and Greece had almost gone to war in a dispute over some rocks (Kardak/Imia) near the Turkish coast (Volkan, 1997b), but what was called "earthquake diplomacy" in many diplomatic circles (Greece itself suffered a smaller earthquake the month following the Turkish disaster) actually initiated a new relationship between the two nations. A closer look at this softening reveals that it was motivated by deep, mostly unremarked, psychological dynamics. The shared aggressive fantasies that accompany enmity have not vanished, but have rather been covered over by an apparent reaction formation: At the large-group level, the generosity provoked by the death of thousands of members of the "enemy" group is fundamentally a defense mechanism against the wish to kill that enemy. But this seemingly negative unconscious motivation does not diminish the reality of the groups' new closeness; the crucial question is whether it can be sublimated. Only time can tell the extent to which Greeks' and Turks' rapprochement can be institutionalized.

Though certain disasters may fall into several categories of shared trauma at once, then, it remains useful to differentiate between the various types because it is only the disaster in which an identifiable enemy group has intentionally inflicted pain, suffering, shame, humiliation, and helplessness on its victims that can trigger a particular large-group identity process. It is only after experiences of war or other ethnic, national, racial, or religious conflict—experiences ranging from terrorist attacks to acts of genocide, from being rendered passive and helpless to being treated as less than human—that the collective trauma exceeds individual PTSD and creates, by transgenerational transmission, certain unconscious tasks for the group's future generations to perform.

During recent decades, the mental health community has learned much about the transgenerational transmission of shared trauma and its relation to the mental health of future generations. Nevertheless, this issue has not received sufficient consideration from those official international organizations and non-governmental organizations (NGOs) that deal with the psychological well-being of refugees, internally displaced individuals, and others who have experienced the horrors of war, the humiliations of warlike conditions, or ethnic cleansing. For example, the official joint manual of the World Health Organization (WHO) and the Office of the United Nations High Commissioner for Refugees (UNHCR; 1996) on the mental health of refugees mentions only crisis intervention methods, relaxation techniques, alcohol and drug problems, and professional conduct toward rape victims. Of course, after a disaster, the crisis situation must take precedence over other considerations, but when the crisis is over, crucial psychological processes continue in full force. The WHO/UNHCR report does not refer at all to the serious issues of societal response and transgenerational transmission following ethnic, national, and religious conflicts, and Dr. Volkan's own professional experience with the WHO and UNHCR at various troubled locations around the world suggests that as of yet, these organizations have neither seriously considered these issues, nor plan to develop strategies for preventive efforts to break the cycle of trauma and pathological transmission.

As suggested in the introduction, our current understanding of the effects of human disaster beyond PTSD owes a great deal to studies of the second and third generations of Holocaust survivors and others directly traumatized under the Third Reich. Needless to say, books examining the historical events of this period through various psychological lenses are legion. Some authors have generalized, on the basis of interviews with hundreds of Holocaust survivors, about the effects of this massive trauma on survivors' mental processes; others have provided detailed clinical studies disproving the supposed uniformity of survivors' psychological responses to the Holocaust. Both sorts of studies have, of course, significantly enriched our understanding of the Nazi period's psychological legacy.

Our aim here, however, is not simply to add to the literature another book on individual psychological problems or adaptations related to personal experiences under the Third Reich. Instead, we focus on the link between clinical work and mental images of shared history; on the relationship between images of ethnic, national, racial, or religious conflicts or genocide and typical intrapsychic developmental conflicts; on the theoretical and practical aspects of how ancestors' traumatic histories influence descendants' identities; and on the therapeutic issues that develop because of these transgenerational transmissions. This chapter briefly examines the history that has brought psychoanalysis to this point.

First Investigations of the Holocaust as Massive Psychic Trauma

Paul Friedman (1949) was among the first psychiatrists to investigate the "deeper psychodynamics of the handful of people who emerged from the camps after liberation" (p. 601). Noting that most of what had been written at that time on the psychological effects of the Holocaust were descriptive accounts of concentration camp experiences written by survivors themselves, he traveled to Cyprus to examine some of the survivors—children as well as adults—being held in a detention center for displaced persons who had sought "illegal" entry into Palestine. Although Friedman's work provided us with valuable insights into these people's defensive and adaptive reactions to their trauma, however, no attempts were made to treat them.

Treatment was available to those survivors who immigrated to the United States, where psychiatric help, psychoanalysis, and other psychotherapies awaited. In the 1960s, more than a decade after Friedman's study, a cascade of psychoanalytic investigations of the internal worlds of Jewish survivors appeared in the literature. Among those working in the United States who grasped some of the significant psychological processes that Jewish survivors had endured was psychoanalyst William Niederland (1961, 1964, 1968), who coined the term *survivor syndrome* to describe the constellation of symptoms brought about by their experiences. Niederland (1968) itemized the characteristics of survivor syndrome as (1) anxiety associated with fears of renewed persecution, sleep disturbances in which "re-run" nightmares play a part, and multiple phobias; (2) disturbed cognition and memory (i.e., amnesia or hyperamnesis), including disorientation in which the present is indistinguishable from the period of persecution; (3) chronic depressive states, covering the spectrum from masochistic character change to psychotic depression, correlated with what Niederland called *survivor guilt*—guilt at having survived the horror that had swept away so many who deserved to live and with whom the survivors often had been closely involved; (4) a tendency to seek isolation, to withdraw into brooding seclusion, with consequent injury to object relations; (5) actual or apparent psychosis, often expressed in paranoid manifestations; (6) altered personal identity, such that the survivor thinks of himself or herself as now "a different person"; (7) chronic tension states, gastrointestinal or cardiovascular disturbances, and what Niederland calls the "typical 'survivor triad': headaches, persistent nightmares, chronic depression, and various other psychosomatic complaints" (p. 313); and (8) a "'walking' or 'shuffling corpse' appearance [that] gives the victim a macabre, shadowy, or ghost-like imprint, difficult to describe, but which seems to be in the nature of an all-pervasive psychological scar on the total personality" (p. 313).

To some extent, Niederland's work led to the presumption that every survivor was obliged to develop psychopathology; it took time for investigators to recognize the variety of adaptations that different survivors made to their massive physical and psychic trauma. Meanwhile, Niederland and other psychoanalysts (among them, Bettelheim, 1960; Chodoff, 1963; de Wind, 1968; Eissler, 1963; Eitinger, 1961, 1964; Fink, 1968; Hoppe, 1966, 1968; Jaffe, 1968; Krystal, 1968; Lorenzer, 1968; Rappaport, 1968; Winnik, 1968) initiated crucial investigations of the various aspects of survivor syndrome and other related intrapsychic processes. In turn, these studies prompted investigators to look at responses to other massive traumas; Lifton (1968), for example, found that survivors of Hiroshima had much in common with the survivors of the Nazi camps.

Overcoming Years of Mass "Denial"

Despite these seminal studies of the 1960s, and despite the fact that by the early 1970s psychoanalytic workshops on survivors' children had begun to take place in earnest (Sonnenberg, 1974; see also Danieli, 1989), a generalized "denial" of the psychological plight of Holocaust survivors strangely persisted—a defense that, astonishingly, extended even to Israel. In a November 25, 1995, story, an Israeli television station reported that even the Jewish state had long neglected the trauma undergone by Holocaust survivors. After their arrival in the 1940s, survivors had been immediately treated for depression and other mental disorders in psychiatric hospitals. Incredibly, however, many of these patients' official files did not even mention that they were Holocaust victims. Israeli psychoanalyst Rafael Moses (1984, 1993) explains that Israeli reaction to certain aspects of the Holocaust was a deep sense of shame. Initially, Israelis who were not directly affected by the tragedy seemed to harbor a wish "not to have these terrible events be true, not to have them touch us, not to be too closely aware of what took place—in other words, a widespread partial use of the mechanism of denial" (Moses and Cohen, 1993, p. 130). Israeli psychologist Judith Stern (Stern, 2000a) argues that after the successful struggle to establish the state of Israel, no image could have been more threatening to the new polity's myth of the fighting (and ultimately victorious) national hero than that of the Holocaust survivor. Significantly, half the Jewish population in Palestine in 1945 had come between 1933 and 1939 and thus had no personal experience of the Holocaust in its full force; as Stern suggests, the survivor could only be understood as a category of "other." Survivors were perceived to have gone "like sheep to the slaughter," Stern reports, in contrast to the *Sabra*, Israeli-born, who knew how to defend themselves. It was far easier for Israelis to identify with the perceived hero than with the victim of total depersonalization whose main "achievement" had been to stay alive in situations of almost inconceivable horror. Indeed, the dichotomy between fighting hero and Holocaust victim became so deeply ingrained that it took many years for the substantial contributions of Holocaust survivors to the Israeli War of Independence to be fully recognized (Yablonka, 1994). Stern (2000b) further suggests that the 1961 trial of Adolf Eichmann represented an important turning point in the process of relinquishing Israeli denial. In the decade following the trial, the second generation, responding to its parents' past experiences of psychological treatment in Israel, began to develop new narratives of the Holocaust experience. Nevertheless, Eva Metzger Brown (1998) estimates that it was 35 years after the end of World War II before things had changed enough among Israelis, and among Jewish people in general, for public denial to dissipate and for survivors to break their conscious silence. By the late 1980s and throughout the 1990s, Israeli mental health professionals were engaged in extensive dialogues with European colleagues about the conditions of survivors and their offspring (Stern, 2000a).

Unsurprisingly, postwar denial in Germany was even more powerful and perhaps more complex. After Adolf Hitler's death and the Allies' installation of a democratic regime in Germany, Germans also wanted to leave the Nazi period untouched, both intellectually and emotionally, despite some public debate of the concept of collective guilt during the Nuremberg war crime trials of 1947. Instead, for the next 20 years, Germans applied their energies mostly to what would become known as the *Wirtschaftswunder* ("economic miracle"). Even the publication of *The Diary of Anne Frank*, the appearance of anti-Semitic graffiti in the early and mid-1960s, and the Eichmann trial did not prompt a national reconsideration of the Third Reich period at an emotional level. As with most societies, it was not until major social and political change forced aside decades-long denials of collective shame and guilt that open examination of the past became possible in Germany. As in the United States and much of the rest of Europe, this major social and political change came in the form of the youth movement of the late 1960s. As resistance to the Vietnam War sanctioned many Americans' interrogation of the United States' supposed moral superiority, so many young Germans began to question the socio-political and military institutions of the postwar Germany in which they had come of age. Moral hypocrisy and militaristic, authoritarian regimes became the ultimate enemies.

In 1967, this growing sense of opposition erupted into the streets when a German student was shot and killed by German police during demonstrations against the visit of Iran's Shah Reza Pahlevi, whom student protestors saw as the representative of an oppressive and authoritarian regime. The demonstrations immediately swelled, rallying against images of any kind of authority. To these activists, behind the public facades of police, judges, and university professors lurked vestiges of the Third Reich. In German universities, students began to disrupt classes, questioning their professors' personal backgrounds, their possible connections with the Nazis, and the relevance of their lectures to current societal issues. Concomitantly, many young people in Germany began to reject traditional patriarchal family values and duties; some began to live in groups known as *Wohngemeinschaften* ("communal living") and championed "free love" as a political statement, saying that "a man who has intercourse twice with the same woman already belongs to the establishment." Thus the "'68 Generation" was born; over the next decade, its antiauthoritarian spirit would evolve in many directions. Many people followed the call by Willy Brandt (Chancellor of Germany from 1969 to 1974) to give up *Außerparlamentarische Opposition* ("Extraparliamentarian Opposition") and instead to begin "the March through the Institutions" in order to reform German society from within. Still others eventually emerged as the Green Party. One group, however, took up weapons, dubbing itself the Rote Armee Fraktion (Red Army Fraction; RAF).

The RAF placed bombs in department stores to protest the exploitation of the Third World and kidnapped powerful and prominent representatives of the "imperialistic system." One of those taken hostage by the RAF in 1977 was the industrial boss Hans Martin Schleyer, seen as a symbol of West Germany's economic elite. Schleyer, who turned out to be a highly disciplined prisoner, a German "type" despised by the kidnappers, was executed after seven weeks when the kidnapping's original aim—to force the release of imprisoned members of the Red Army Fraction fighters—failed. Twenty years later, Heinrich Breloer (1997) described this event as the face-off of the "bad Nazi father" and the "good" sons (p. 129); in an interview for a documentary film about the "seven weeks of civil war" entitled *Todesspiel* ("Death Game"), RAF kidnapper Peter-Jürgen Boock concurred with this analogy (p. 9). Over the weeks that Schleyer was held, however, a remarkable phenomenon emerged. Gradually, the Red Army Fraction kidnappers became increasingly militant and began to use quasi-Nazi terminology such as *Volksgefängnis* ("people's prison"), *Gefangener der Bewegung* ("prisoner of the movement"), and *Volksgericht* ("people's trial"). Breloer asserts that within those seven weeks, the kidnappers had arrived at "a place that they never wanted to arrive at: in the country [Nazi Germany] of their parents" (p. 125). Like their Nazi ancestors, Breloer adds, the members of the Red Army Fraction behaved with discipline, self-righteousness, grandiosity, and emotional coldness. To us, it appears that those who declared their rage toward all "oppressors" themselves incorporated elements of Nazism.

The 1970s, the maturation period of the "'68 Generation," saw what Margarete Mitscherlich-Nielsen describes as a flood of books and movies on Hitler. Indeed, by 1979, she could plausibly claim that Germans no longer objected to digging in their Nazi past. She believed, however, that Germans' intellectual preoccupation with factual material about Hitler's childhood, developmental years, and rise to power was mainly a defense. We think that what Mitscherlich-Nielsen saw as defensive preoccupation might also have served as a necessary step in overcoming that defensiveness; what Hitler had launched was so monstrous that Germans first needed intellectually to understand him—as a man, with a childhood and life struggles, who had grown up to lead his nation into horrible crimes—before they could develop an emotional comprehension of the past and of their own involvement in and responsibility for it. In psychoanalytic terms, we believe that the Germans needed to integrate their idealized Hitler with their monster Hitler in order to integrate their own collective self-representation.

The reunification of East and West Germany was another major political change that, as Dieter Ohlmeier (1991) declared, was also a major psychological event, prompting a new wave of renegotiations with the Nazi past. Among these renegotiations was the "Nazi skinhead" movement in Germany, a maladaptive manifestation of shame and guilt derivations (Rosenthal, 1997; Streeck-Fischer, 1999). Indeed, investigation of the Nazi skinhead phenomenon itself became a vehicle for lifting more general societal denial. As Ohlmeier suggests, psychoanalytic considerations of German reunification finally evoked "questions of a psychology of the Germans, and the necessity of a psychohistorical reflection of the Germans since 1933," a charge that has been taken up by a number of people in the German psychiatric and psychological community. In August 1998, a group of five German psychiatrists and psychologists (two of them Jewish) organized a major meeting in Düsseldorf called "*Das Ende der Sprachlosigkeit?*" ("The End of Speechlessness?"). Also attended by psychoanalysts, this interdisciplinary meeting confronted both intellectually and emotionally the "speechlessness" that has surrounded the Third Reich in Germany (see chapter 9). Unlike the "'68 Generation," the Germans in this group wondered not only what their fathers did during the Third Reich, but also what their parents had transmitted to them—even when the parents themselves remained "silent" about the Nazi period. The question mark at the end of the conference title expressed their doubts about the complete end of that silence. In a related effort, the München Arbeitskreis für Psychoanalyse (MAP; Munich Study Group for Psychoanalysis) has planned a five-year series of workshops to help psychoanalytic supervisors increase their awareness of the Nazi period's influence in their patients' psychopathology and related technical issues.

Large-Group Historical Trauma Across Generational Boundaries

Through hundreds and hundreds of publications (many of which we will cite in the course of this book), conferences, group meetings, and works of art, we know that in spite of the fact that the traumatic period of the Third Reich has now been over for more than half a century, its influence still reverberates not only in the minds of the original victims, but also in those of subsequent generations. Indeed, only in the past several decades have clinicians begun to understand the extent to which the effects of this historical trauma have transcended its immediate survivors and perpetrators. Only through in-depth psychological studies of the second, and in some cases third, generations of survivors have clinicians become aware that images of the Holocaust have passed the pathogenic influence of Nazi atrocities across generational psychic boundaries—though the mechanisms of such transmissions have awaited further investigation.

Through these many studies, we have learned that the supposed uniformity of the survivor syndrome and of the content transmitted to subsequent generations is highly questionable. First of all, as Henri Parens (1999) points out, the Holocaust was not a single massive event: Different survivors had different experiences. Some survivors had been in labor camps and others in extermination camps; some were children during the Nazi period, some adults; some had come from dysfunctional families, and some had developed good internalized object relations prior to experiencing trauma. Careful psychoanalytic studies of survivors—such as those provided by Deborah J. Terry (1984), Anna Ornstein (1985), Judith Kestenberg and Ira Brenner (1996), Milton Jucovy (1998), and Henri Parens (1999)—clearly document that the experiences of directly affected persons were highly individualized. Even when a group of people shares the same massive trauma, long-term adaptation will have different outcomes in different individuals. These investigators further conclude that even though the individual's ego strength and internalized object relations prior to the trauma were indeed a crucial determinant of survivors' adaptation to the post-Nazi world, "massive, severe, and cumulative trauma may be the most significant determinant in the appearance of late symptoms, despite pre-Holocaust predispositions" (Jucovy, 1998, p. 32).

What survivors transmitted of their experiences to their offspring has thus proven quite variable as well. Moreover, what those in the next generations have done with what has been passed on to them has proven to depend to a large extent upon other elements of their family backgrounds; developmental conflicts; feelings of guilt, ambivalence, shame, or murderous rage; and so on. Although not everyone to whom elements of survivors' experiences have been transmitted responds maladaptively, some do respond with psychopathology. Because the patients whose cases we report in this book exhibited symptoms, maladaptive character traits, and/or difficulties in object relations, our emphasis here is necessarily on pathological outcomes. What we can generalize is that after shared massive trauma, some transgenerational transmission of its images does occur, becoming intertwined with the *core identity* (an individual's subjective experiences of his or her inner sameness while sharing certain characteristics with others [Erikson, 1956]) and *self-representation* (the metapsychological reconstruction of an individual's self-concept) of each member of subsequent generations in the groups for which the trauma is a historical legacy.

In order to examine how the transgenerational transmission of shared massive trauma takes place, it is first necessary to review the relationship between generations more generally. The following chapter explains the role that significant others—that is, parents, siblings, teachers—play in a child's mental development.

2

The Role of Others
IN MENTAL DEVELOPMENT

THE CRUCIAL ROLE THAT PERSONS and things and their images or representations—called "objects" in psychoanalysis—play in mental development has been widely acknowledged in psychoanalysis since its inception. Before elaborating our understanding of that role further, however, let us distinguish between a *representation* and an *image*. After developing the capacity to differentiate the self from others, a person's ego develops an "image" of the other—and a corresponding "image" of the self—whenever that person interacts with another. Embodied in these images are individuals' wishes, affects, and perceptions surrounding the objects, as well as their defenses against them; thus an individual can hold manifold and varied images of the same object at different times. By "representation," on the other hand, we mean a relatively permanent aggregate of such images of an object, a mosaic constructed by the ego from the individual's multiple real and fantasy experiences with that object. Such an aggregate of images, some of which are mostly conscious and some of which are mostly unconscious, comprises, for example, a child's "mother representation," which may or may not correspond to the child's actual mother in any given respect. A mental representation is, in a sense, analogous to a cast of characters in a theatrical production, only some of whom are on stage at any particular moment. Thus, when it is said that individuals transmit their traumatized "self-representation," it is not truly their *representation* that is being transmitted, but their traumatized *image*. We are aware that some massive traumas may affect the whole mosaic of images; nevertheless, for our purposes, *image* will be the more specific term, *representation* the global.

The Roles of Objects in Early Mental Development

Sigmund Freud's "Mourning and Melancholia" (1917b), a transitional paper between his topographical and structural models of the mind, contains some of his most fertile thinking on the role that external reality, in the form of object loss, plays in mental life. When a love object is lost, the shadow of its mental representation (to use the terminology outlined previously) falls on the mourner's self-representation. Thus, the representation of the object already present in the internal world of the mourner becomes exaggerated, and an intense relationship develops between the mourner's self-representation and the internalized object-representation of the lost person. The work of mourning and its outcome depend upon what the mourner does with this internal relationship with the representation of the lost person. In "normal" mourning, mourners selectively identify with the "good" images of the lost object and, in so doing, enrich their self-representation through healthy identification with these images. In melancholia, mourners also form an identification—but this time with both "good" and "bad" image-elements in their ambivalently held representation of the lost object. This melancholic identification turns mourners' internal worlds into battlegrounds where they struggle with their guilt-ridden wish to "kill" the representation, on the one hand, and their wish to "save and repair" it, on the other. (We will discuss these and other possible outcomes for the work of mourning further in chapter 5.)

This replacement of object-cathexis by identification, Freud also discovered, is not only characteristic of "normal" mourning or of melancholia but also, in fact, of mental development in general: "We have come to understand that this kind of substitution has a great share in determining the form taken by the ego and that it makes an essential contribution towards building up what is called its 'character,'" he writes (Freud, 1923, p. 28). Ego development, then, is based in the history of the child's earliest internalized object relations and is therefore " . . . a precipitate of abandoned object cathexes" (Freud, 1923, p. 29). Of course, Freud's concept of the superego involves combining identification with objects and their images as well, particularly during the oedipal phase. These writings show that Freud understood that the mental apparatus does not evolve in a vacuum, but rather is molded by early internalized object relations—the vestiges of which are apparent in the very form and character of an individual's psychic organization as an adult.

It is important to note that Freud studied the significance of objects primarily from the vantage of the child's internal world, theorizing that a child's object-images or representations are fundamentally shaped by what the child externalizes and projects upon them; for example, the image of a father might be transformed into that of a dangerous castrator by an oedipal-stage son's projection of his own aggression onto that image. That is, Freud focused on what children put into their images of objects from their internal worlds rather than on what was put into children from others' self-concepts. Melanie Klein (1946) carried this sort of thinking to an extreme. Though she acknowledged that there is a reality "out there," she stressed almost exclusively the psychic importance of objects modified by the child's projections—especially projections of death instinct derivatives—and the child's identification with these modified objects (*projective identification*). Thus she wrote about mental development as if it occurred without interactions with a *real* external world.

As time has passed since Freud's work, researchers have come to appreciate much more fully the complexity of the reciprocal projective-introjective processes that transpire between children (or regressed adults) and their environment. It is beyond the scope of this chapter to review the various theories that emphasize the role of objects in the outer world in the development of a child's self-concept, but we will note just a few examples: Erik Erikson's (1954, 1956) description of identity-formation as the ego's successful synthesis of "social realit[ies]" (p. 168) with postadolescent drive organization; Donald Winnicott's (1960) explication of the "facilitating environment"; Hans Leowald's (1960) observation that as children internalize aspects of their mothers, they internalize parents' image of themselves at the same time; and Edith Jacobson (1964), Margaret Mahler (1968), and Otto Kernberg's (1975, 1980) systematizations of internalized object-relations development and the role of objects in that process.

More recent studies have suggested a biological foundation for the psychological permeability between infants and their mothers. In Kuopio, Finland, researchers focusing on maternal responses to audiotapes of crying infants have established that a mother *physiologically* responds differently to her own child's cry than to that of any other child. Johannes Lehtonen and other Finnish researchers are also researching infants' physiological responses to various nursing experiences with analogous results, suggesting that there is a "hole" between infants and their mothers through which the psychobiological elements that create the special relationship between the two individuals flow (Lehtonen et al., 1998; Lehtonen, 1999).

Clinicians have also observed how mental contents can pass between regressed adults. Harold Searles (1959) long ago described the phenomenon of "driving the other crazy"; by unconscious mechanisms, the psychotic aspect of one person is passed to another so that the first individual can maintain the illusion of getting rid of highly disruptive, troubling mental content. Sheldon Heath (1991) invokes the Kleinian concept of projective identification to explain a similar phenomenon among therapists who became depressed through contact with their depressed patients: "part of the self is put unconsciously into another person, so that there is the feeling of being in the other's psyche in various ways" (p. 70). Of course, less dramatic examples of this phenomenon can be observed in more routine clinical work. Because psychoanalysis initially emphasized how the child's instinctual drives shape the images of intimate objects, however, investigators have usually ignored what children have internalized into their representational world uncontaminated, or relatively uncontaminated, by their own externalizations and projections. Consequently, we believe it is crucial to examine more fully the significance of the child's objects in their own right.

As more and more was learned about the roles of objects in the evolution of a child's mind, then, modern psychoanalytic research (Ainsworth, Bell, and Stayton, 1974; Brazelton, Koslowski, and Main, 1974; Emde, 1988a, 1988b, and 1991; Greenspan, 1989; and Stern, 1985) also began to inform us of the inborn psychobiological potentials of the infant. Before proceeding further, however, we should state how difficult—if not impossible—it is to tease apart the child's inherited psychobiological potentials from the role of the parents and caretakers in stimulating these potentials. What Veikko Tähkä (1988, 1993) called the fundamental mental function potentials, such as perception and memory, develop in an average expectable environment (Hartmann, 1950) during activities such as nursing at the mother's breast. The evolution of complicated mental function potentials, such as integration of opposing self- and object-images and tolerance for ambivalence, however, requires an intimate, attuned relationship with the maternal object (such potentials are enriched when the child moves from dyadic to triadic [oedipal] and then on to multiple object relations). Since they can unfold only in the context of more complex object relationships, they are more vulnerable to environmental deficiencies and complications (Tähkä, 1988, 1993). Psychic structure formation, then, depends heavily upon optimal maternal psychic availability in the earliest months of an infant's life and throughout the child's formative years.

Earlier researchers of mother–child interactions such as René Spitz (1957, 1965) and Margaret Mahler (1968), as well as more recent investigators such as Robert Emde (1988a, 1988b, 1991) and Stanley Greenspan (1989), have shown that most infants' psychobiological potentials "hatch" when caretaker–child experiences serve as their incubator; without an object and its nurturing images, these potentials fail to emerge. Volkan (1997a) provides a list of elements, some originating in the child and some in the mother or other primary caretaker, that coalesce during child–caretaker interactions to shape the child's mental development. The child's genetic/biological "givens" and the conjunction of the mother/caretaker's temperament and activities and those of the child should be considered the "first elements" of this mixture, but the amalgam of significant elements also includes the intensity of the child's drive derivatives, including affects; growth-stimulating and growth-inhibiting external events; fixation-producing traumas; the mother/caretaker's support or interference with the child's transitional objects/phenomena and transitional space; available and unavailable identifications; various ego functions (later superego functions); and cultural and educational variables. As children move up in their development from a dyadic object relationship to a triadic (oedipal) one, and then to multiple internalized object relationships, the interactions between children and various significant other people in their environment enrich this mixture of elements. The mix of "ingredients" that ultimately accumulates will determine not only the nature of children's mental development—that is, their ego functions and personality organization—but also the nature of children's core identity formations as well as the evolution, integration, and cohesion of their self-representation.

Though Volkan mentions "cultural and educational" variables in a general way, the parents' (or other significant persons') mental representation of the specific historical experiences of the large group to which they belong is not among the elements he lists. This book adds to that list of crucial variables the mental representation of large-group shared history to which each individual child is heir.

Two Types of Large-Group History

When we speak of history here, we are not referring to a person's own unique "historical" development—for example, being born into a poor family, having siblings, finishing high school, becoming rich as an adult, getting married, becoming a parent, being involved in a car accident, and so on. Nor are we speaking of "official history" as chronicled by scholars, though we are interested in many of the same events that engage historians: experiences that are shared by the thousands or millions of people who are affiliated with a large-group identity.

To clarify the type of mental representation of history that is meant here, representations affected by a large group's historical experiences will be divided into two categories: survivors and their descendants. A survivor, either as a child or as an adult, is psychologically injured to a greater or lesser extent as a result of personally experiencing a historical event such as a war; the mental representation of the event is not something that is passed into this individual's mind by someone else. For example, those living in Kuwait during the Iraqi seven-month occupation in 1990, the 300,000 internally displaced persons (IDPs) in the Republic of Georgia after the Georgian–Abkhazian and Georgian–South Ossetian conflicts of 1991–1992, the people of Sarajevo who endured the long siege and bombing of their city by the Serbs in 1992, and the Kosovar Albanians driven out of Kosovo by Serbs in 1999 were all survivors of large-group trauma. Such traumas affect a society on many levels. Those who fight or are tortured, raped, humiliated, or displaced from their homes and those who experience significant material or emotional losses are obviously most directly and massively traumatized and may require clinical treatment. Those members of the group who are not personally traumatized are still subject to less direct, but nevertheless powerful, psychological, social, political, and economic effects, for the losses and physical destruction are also experienced as attacks on an ethnic or national group's pride.

It is important to note that these forms of indirect traumatization are unique to experiences of trauma caused by an enemy group; they usually do not characterize responses to man-made disasters such as Three Mile Island or Chernobyl, or to natural disasters such as earthquakes, tornadoes, and typhoons. As was discussed in chapter 1, natural or accidental disasters should be differentiated from those massive traumas due to ethnic or other large-group conflicts, which initiate a number of specific shared psychological processes for the members of the groups involved. First, when a large group's conflict with a neighboring large group becomes inflamed, the bonding between members belonging to the same large group intensifies, resulting in an exaggeration of the usual rituals of differentiation between one large group and another. Indeed, under stressful conditions, members' investments in their large-group identity may become more important than their individual identities (Volkan, 1997b, 1999a, 1999b, 1999c). When two ethnic groups are in "hot" conflict, the usual rituals are intensified to the point that they become the two prescriptions governing relationships between people in each group: (1) maintain one's large-group identity separate from the identity of the enemy so that any commonalities they may share are erased; and (2) keep a psychological border between the two large groups at any cost. It is because of this phenomenon that "minor differences" (Freud 1917a, 1930) between neighboring groups develop into major political issues, since "minor" differences become the last markers by which to maintain that boundary. When large groups are not "the same," each can externalize and project more effectively its unwanted aspects on the enemy group, up to and including dehumanizing (Bernard, Ottenberg, and Redl, 1973) that enemy. Anything that contravenes these two mandates induces massive anxiety, and large groups may feel entitled to do anything to preserve the differences they ensure, thereby perpetuating hostilities. Again, when one large group victimizes another one, those who are traumatized do not turn to "fate" or "God," as victims of natural disasters often do, to understand and assimilate the effects of the tragedy. Instead, they often become possessed by their sense of rage and entitlement to revenge.

But these feelings oscillate with helplessness, shame, humiliation, and victimization. Such internal turmoil blocks the evolution of certain psychological processes that the victims need to go through in order to assimilate their tragedy and to accept the changes caused by it—and among these psychological processes is the work of mourning (Freud, 1917b). Humans are obliged to mourn their losses and changes in life; mourning allows us to accept that a loss or change has occurred. Without it, people remain trapped in the dilemma of whether to accept the tragedy and to adjust to life after it, metaphorically remaining hidden in the basement after the tornado has passed over and fair weather has returned. An individual (or a society) traumatized deliberately by "others" has a tendency to "remain in the basement"; the sense of shame, humiliation, guilt, and helplessness may become internalized, complicating the survivors' individual fates.

As we have suggested, the degree to which a war or warlike situation affects individuals within a traumatized large group depends upon such variables as the actual nature of the historical event itself, the individual's external conditions, and their previous level of psychic organization; the mental representation of the large group's traumatic experience becomes intertwined with its individual members' existing psychological processes. When the current historical trauma is over, survivors may exhibit symptoms of what is known in psychiatry as post-traumatic stress disorder (PTSD), the traumatized victim's tendency to repeat aspects of the traumatic experience compulsively in thoughts about current events, interpersonal relations, daydreams, and nightmares. For the survivor, persons in the present become identified with those who were involved in the original trauma, including victimizer, victim, and wished-for helper. Thoughts, affects, and behavior that occurred at the time of the trauma may be repeated without clear conscious awareness of their association with the ordeal. Clinical studies (Horowitz, 1986; Thomson, 2000) have clearly demonstrated the tendency of this phenomenon to recur again and again without therapeutic intervention.

Though in this book we refer to historical events that directly influenced or traumatized individuals and thereby created traumatized large groups, the mental representation of history that we will focus on belongs primarily to the second category of individuals affected by a shared historical trauma: the descendant of the trauma survivor. In descendants, the mental representation of a historical event is passed into the developing core identity and self-representation of individuals through their early interactions with their parents or other caretakers. We concentrate, therefore, on representations of historical events that occurred either before individuals who possess those representations were born or when they were babies, and about which they could therefore have developed no formed mentation. The type of large-group history on which this book focuses, then, is the history of collective indirect experience.

As this discussion suggests, large-group historical traumas are thus not simply comprised of static, shared conscious memories of the event. Rather, they are highly dynamic complexes of recollections, fantasies, affects, wishes, and defenses (i.e., mental representations), whose influences are transmitted from generation to generation. Persisting in the minds of members consciously and unconsciously, these complexes have long life-spans—in some cases, hundreds of years. It is this complex of mental representation that is passed to future generations who, as "carriers," must cope with the unmastered psychological tasks given to them by their ancestors.

Before exploring how representations of historical experience initiate history-related unconscious fantasies in an individual, it is necessary to understand the mechanisms by which such mental representations are passed from generation to generation. Chapter 3 now turns to the various types of transgenerational transmission.

3

Varieties of TRANSGENERATIONAL TRANSMISSION

THE PHENOMENON OF TRANSGENERATIONAL TRANSMISSION has long been known to psychoanalysts. The pioneering work of Anna Freud and Dorothy Burlingham (1942) examined the unconscious affective "messages" passed between mothers and their children during the German bombing of London in World War II. Subsequent investigators working with regressed patients added important insights into the process by which a mother's anxiety becomes her child's; Harry S. Sullivan's (1962) work on schizophrenia in the 1960s emphasized this affective flow between a mother and her offspring. Our own clinical work repeatedly illustrates the crucial fluidity of psychic borders between parent/caregiver and child; over and over we see that not only parents/caregivers' anxiety, depression, and other affects, but also their unconscious fantasies, perceptions, and expectations of the external world—including those related to the child—can pass into the child's developing sense of self.

In the clinical setting, it is sometimes possible to detect, in individuals' symptoms or object relations, the derivatives of unconscious fantasies that have been passed into their psychic organization. Studies on transsexualism (Apprey, 1993b; Volkan and Berent, 1976; Volkan and Greer, 1995) provide an example of this type of transgenerational transmission. These studies clearly demonstrate that although transsexual persons believe that they have male or female gender identities incongruent with biological reality, children's "incongruent" gender identities have been "created" in their parents' minds—in other words, these are the parents' fantasies—and then passed on to the children, who experience those identities as real. Condensed with other crucial psychological constellations, such as depression in the parents, these experiences produce in the minds of the offspring the compensatory unconscious fantasies of sex-change as a means by which to please parents and save them from their depression—hence transsexuals' familiar refrain that they are "trapped in the body of the wrong sex."

Volkan and As'ad Masri's (1989) study of transsexual Carla and her mother provides an illustration. Carla, calling herself Carlos when she began work with Volkan and Masri, was born while her father was away on military assignment in a distant country. While awaiting her husband's return, Carla's mother became depressed and sexually "hungry." To allay this "hunger," she daydreamed about affairs with various movie stars. While pregnant with Carla, furthermore, the mother imagined that her new baby would be a boy, who, unlike her husband, would satisfy her libidinal hunger. Several months after Carla's birth, her mother began to masturbate, placing the baby between her legs as if the child were a penis. When she took Carla for a stroll in the baby carriage, she covered her up as one wraps a male child so as not to exhibit his penis in public, and she often referred to her infant daughter as "he." At one point during the study, Carla's mother mused: "This may sound silly, but is it possible that I could have transmitted my thoughts about this to my daughter?" Indeed, she had. Carla experienced her mother's fantasized object-image (satisfying penis) as a real element in her own self-representation and thus subjectively considered herself "a male in the body of a female." So concrete was this sense that Carla imagined that if she could unzip her skin as one does a sports jacket, she would find a penis beneath it. She sought surgical sex "reassignment" to actualize her mother's wish for her to be a baby/penis and thereby to rescue her mother from despair.

It is also well-known that psychic borders are permeable in a relationship between two adults—a grown child and a parent or unrelated individuals—when they relate to one another under regressed states. As an example, let us look at a relationship between mother and child among the Georgian internally displaced persons (IDPs) living in Tbilisi Sea, a former resort area near a huge man-made lake in the suburbs of the Republic of Georgia's capital. Marli and her three children were among those dwelling in one of three former hotels housing 3,000 of the 300,000 Georgian IDPs who still remained homeless when Dr. Volkan visited the area in 1998. As Doruna—Marli's 16-year-old youngest child—and Dr. Volkan talked alone on the cluttered balcony of the hotel room that had been the family's cramped home since the wars between Georgians and Abkhazians and between Georgians and South Ossetians in the early 1990s, the young woman told Dr. Volkan that she and her mother kept their worries to themselves. As is typical within refugee families, silence was frequently their mode of communication, as if talking about painful things would hurt the other and therefore must be avoided. Nevertheless, as again is typical, Doruna knew of her mother's recurring yet unspoken worry: Each night, as the mother herself told Dr. Volkan in a separate conversation, Marli went to bed wondering how she would be able to buy food the next day. While Doruna was telling Dr. Volkan this story, Marli, who had grown thinner since becoming a refugee, came to the balcony and asked Dr. Volkan to "do something" about her daughter—the girl would not exercise, her mother complained, and was getting fat. "Please, as a physician, tell her to exercise," Marli pleaded.

Dr. Volkan suggested that Marli ask Doruna whether she were aware of her mother's daily anxiety about being able to feed her children. After Marli and Doruna talked together, Dr. Volkan counseled Marli that Doruna "had" to stay overweight, at least for now; by being overweight, he believed, the daughter was trying to tell her mother, "Don't worry about finding food for your children. As you can see, I am more than well-fed." Furthermore, Dr. Volkan recommended that mother and daughter try to share their worries directly through open communication rather than indirectly through bodily expression. When Dr. Volkan visited Marli and Doruna six months later, he was delighted to note that the young woman had lost weight; both she and her mother attributed the emergence of a more physically healthy Doruna to his diagnosis and counsel. During subsequent visits over the next two years, Dr. Volkan found Doruna still slim and healthy.

This brief anecdote illustrates the transgenerational transmission of a mother's worry to her daughter and the daughter's attempt to "repair" and reassure her mother: a task given by a person in one generation to a person in another without either of them being fully conscious of it. Affect, worry, and parental unconscious or semiconscious fantasies are not the only things that can be transmitted transgenerationally, though; adults can also deposit an already-formed self- or internalized object-image with its associated affects into the developing self-representation of a child on the mostly unconscious belief that there it can be "safe," that there the resolution of the conflict with which it is associated can be postponed until a future time, or that the recipient of the image—the child—will resolve the conflict.

The Tasks Associated with Transgenerationally Transmitted Self- or Object-Images

Robert Zuckerman and Vamık Volkan (1988) report the case of a woman with a congenital spinal deformity who, unable either to reverse this trauma or to mourn the lack of a more functional body, passed on her "defective" body image to her son. The spinal deformity had become condensed in the mother's mind with psychosexual and other developmental difficulties. In an unconscious attempt to "cure" herself, she shepherded the boy to physicians, insisting that they treat his "deformed spine," even though in reality his spine was normal. The boy himself came to believe in his own deformity and collaborated with his mother in a search for a repaired body. It had fallen to the boy to deal with his mother's traumatized image and to accomplish for her what she was never able to accomplish for herself: to fulfill the wish for a healthier body or to mourn the lack of it. He had become a reservoir for a traumatized body image from a previous generation and was burdened with the psychological tasks that rightfully belonged to that previous generation.

Dr. Greer treated a young woman, Lili, whose mother had become pregnant as a result of being raped by a man of another race when she was in her late adolescence. Because of her religious beliefs, she carried the baby to term and gave it up for adoption; later, she married Lili's father. Unable either to resolve her guilt for giving up her first baby or to work through the trauma of the rape, Lili's mother passed her traumatized self-image, as well as internalized object-images involved in the trauma, to her daughter—who, in turn, began to reenact her mother's drama as she reached late adolescence.

For years, Lili's mother had told her daughter that she "just knew" that Lili would become pregnant out of wedlock. As Lili grew older and appeared to be more interested in her studies than in boys, however, her mother suggested that she needed to learn to "flirt" if she was ever going to snare a man and get married. But, her mother admonished, Lili should take birth control pills so as not to get pregnant. Around this same time, her mother disclosed to Lili the story of the rape and her first child. The mother's mixed messages about sexuality reflected her simultaneous wish to kill her first child and the guilt she felt both for having this wish and for having given up the child for adoption.

Soon after Lili began treatment, it began to appear to Dr. Greer that she was "under the spell" of her parent's past. A single dream indicated the depth of what had been deposited in her. In the dream, Lili found herself alone in a house, terrified of a man with a gun whom she could see just outside the window. She tried to close the blinds, but they were too narrow to cover the whole window. As she described the scenario: "He would kill me if I did not do exactly as he demanded, so I had no alternative but to submit to rape." In the dream, as she awaited the inevitable, she suddenly recalled having been raped earlier in her life, feeling intense shame as she thought about the earlier rape and her passive compliance with the imminent one. In the dream, she desperately wanted to tell her mother about the earlier rape "so she would finally know the truth, but Mom was nowhere to be found." In reality, though, Lili had never been raped: It was the image of Lili's mother, the one who had actually been raped, that was appearing *as an image of Lili* in Lili's own dream. When Lili associated in response to the dream, she expressed surprise that she had made no effort to escape, something she "knew" she would have done if she were ever really attacked. She had always "accused victims of not fighting back and giving in too soon." Indeed, as she associated, she even questioned whether her mother had been raped, because her mother "did not present it as a violent act." Not long after having this dream, Lili began to take leisurely strolls through a park where women had recently been assaulted. She now seemed so thoroughly under the influence of her parent's victimized self-image that Dr. Greer, concerned for her safety, advised his patient to stop this dangerous behavior and instead to explore the meanings of the impulse behind it.

Over the next several sessions, it gradually became possible to suggest to the patient that she had become a reservoir for her mother's traumatized image and was under a compulsion to repeat her mother's past. Shortly thereafter, however, Lili became involved with a young man of the same race as the man who raped her mother and began to have unprotected sex with him. She professed to be deeply in love with him and repudiated all of Dr. Greer's efforts to discuss the possible connection between this liaison and the reservoir-function he had proposed in their earlier therapeutic work. It was not long before the patient announced that she was pregnant. She agonized over what to do: Should she have an abortion, give the baby up for adoption, or raise it as a single parent? This conscious struggle was condensed with what she fantasized her own mother to have gone through years earlier upon finding herself pregnant by the man who had raped her. In a sense, Lili had a task, unconsciously given to her by her mother through mixed messages about sexuality, to bear a child to replace the one her mother had given away. But Lili also "knew" that her mother wished to get rid of that baby. Once she was able to free herself from her parent's dilemma through therapeutic work, she chose to have an abortion and to break off the relationship with her boyfriend.

Dr. Volkan and Dr. Ast (1994) have previously reported the case of Peter, whose stepfather—who had played a significant role in his upbringing—was a survivor of the infamous Bataan Death March during World War II. After surrendering to the Japanese, some 70,000 American and Filipino prisoners were forced to march approximately 63 miles of the distance from Bataan to Camp O'Donnell, with no food, water, or protection from the scorching sun. During the march, the prisoners were also beaten and humiliated by their Japanese captors; those who were too sick to march or who straggled behind the column in the sweltering heat were summarily killed. Within a period of six weeks after the march, 11,600 Americans and unknown thousands of Filipinos died. Those who survived, including Peter's stepfather, remained in the O'Donnell prison camp for some years.

Peter's stepfather's period of imprisonment could only have been harrowing. Arnold Bocksel (1991), who was a prisoner himself during World War II, describes the conditions that existed in a similar Japanese prison camp in the Philippines:

> Flies were another enemy we encountered in prison camp. Droves and droves of them flitting from the open latrines to our mess kits, our hands, faces, and every part of our exposed bodies. We were constantly shooing them away. It was pitiful to see a dying man, face and hands encrusted with those goddamn flies, and be oblivious to their presence. (p. 32)

Flies, indeed, were one of the primary causes for the rampant spread of dysentery among the prisoners, the disease that was responsible for so many deaths, especially in prisoners' first years of incarceration. Prisoners caught trying to escape this misery were executed, often by public decapitation. Remaining prisoners, who looked like cadavers themselves, were assigned to carry the bodies of those who had died or been executed the day before to a large ditch dug as a mass grave. "The bodies," Bocksel writes, "were thrown into the large pits, one on top of the other. In the rainy season, legs, arms, and other parts would protrude from the ground and had to be recovered with dirt" (p. 34; see also Stewart, 1956).

As far as we could ascertain from Peter's remarks, his stepfather seemed to have led a "normal" life after being repatriated at the end of the war. As would soon become apparent, however, he appeared "normal" because he had externalized his traumatized self-image and associated internalized object-images—and had externalized them perhaps most significantly onto the young Peter.

Soon after entering Peter's life, the veteran built a multistoried purple martin house for the garden of the home in which the family would remain for the next several decades: Perched atop a pole firmly set in concrete, the birdhouse turned out to be a quite tangible externalization of the stepfather's "imprisoned" self-image and associated object-images and affects. For decades it was full of birds that, in due course, laid and hatched eggs and launched fledglings. Peter's stepfather carefully painted numbers on each of the many "apartments" he had built for bird families to occupy; over the years, he meticulously banded the legs of all the fledglings, marking each with the number of its family "apartment." If a baby bird had an untimely fall from the martin house, he would then know to which "apartment" it belonged and could return it safely, since a fledgling rescued by a human hand and returned to the wrong nest would be rejected and die.

In psychoanalysis, Peter came to understand that in constructing and tending the birdhouse, his stepfather had built a new and benign version of the Japanese prison camp, where there had been constant restraint and regulation, ceaseless horror and death. In the new version, no occupant would be allowed to die. Unlike in the prison, intervention in individual lives would only be benevolent. The stepfather had symbolically reversed his past reality, inventing a new fate for himself and his comrades by creating a new camp in which all (his injured self-image and his internalized images of his prison mates) would be safe and happy.

Besides the purple martin house, Peter's developing identity and self-representation were the principal depository for his stepfather's externalized injured self. When the stepfather came into his life, the one-year-old Peter had been obese, a direct result of being dominated by his mother and grandmother. After her first husband left just after Peter's birth, the mother was depressed and angry, and this anger had apparently been transferred to her son. Abetted by her own mother, she literally forced little Peter's food down his throat, profoundly inhibiting the boy's efforts to develop his own autonomy. Indeed, in a sense,

Peter was in a "prison" himself; while in analysis, he dreamed about his childhood environment by seeing himself alone in a space dome—isolated under the control of these two women.

The stepfather must have unconsciously perceived this correspondence between the frustrated little boy and his own helpless self-image as a prisoner of war, a resemblance that made Peter a suitable repository for the traumatized images and affects that were too horrific for the stepfather to acknowledge and to assimilate into his own self-representation. The stepfather had to ensure that his traumatized self- and object-images externalized into Peter's identity and self-representation would not return to him, so he also encouraged in the young Peter a defensive self-image; this Peter now needed in order to combat the injured self-image that had absorbed his stepfather's traumatized images. The stepfather introduced the child to guns and encouraged the adolescent Peter to develop a muscular body. The message being sent to Peter was that it is better to hunt than to be hunted: better to be a powerful, armed aggressor than the target of another's aggression.

As Peter grew older, this powerful self-image dominated his conscious mental life and activities, though his own "imprisoned" self persisted unmodified, split off. Peter was a hunter, but not a sportsman; he often turned to hunting when his dominant identity was threatened. Periodically, in a state of anxiety, he would charter a helicopter, fly over a herd of deer, and slaughter as many as he could with a machine gun. The animals that Peter killed, particularly deer, came to symbolize Peter's "imprisoned" childhood self-image condensed with his stepfather's helpless images. In a memorable dream in the fourth year of his analysis, Peter saw himself " . . . with a man who was handsome. I saw red foxes running along a valley. When I pointed out the foxes, he pointed to another animal, a disfigured deer with thick, clumsy legs and no horns." Peter identified the red foxes as his mother and grandmother, because when he was a child these women used to wear red bikinis; furthermore, he had repeatedly witnessed his mother's menstrual flow. The handsome man in the dream represented his stepfather, who, as the strong oedipal father Peter wished for, could conquer Peter's "suffocating women." The disfigured deer represented Peter's image of himself as a castrated (hornless), ungainly boy. Little Peter was searching for a strong oedipal father with whom to identify, in order to escape the smothering "prison" run by his mother and grandmother.

As an adult, Peter extended his investment in his conscious self-image as dominant and powerful by becoming professionally involved in the military-industrial complex, and he and his stepfather continued to hunt together. Peter persisted in killing animals in a savage and malignant manner, but on the walls of a special large room of his home, Peter hung trophies of his hunts so skillfully prepared through taxidermy that they looked alive. Among the many meanings and functions of Peter's work in taxidermy that Dr. Volkan and Dr. Ast discerned was this: The results of this hobby embodied the stepfather's imprisoned self-image surrounded by images of his dead prison-camp comrades. Peter sometimes sat in his special room for hours gazing at the trophies, symbolically (but unconsciously) taking his stepfather's place and admiring, as it were, his work of resurrection. Because Peter took such pains to make the trophies look "alive," he had created the illusion that he had repaired his stepfather's self- and object-images.

After five years of analysis Peter began to get well and to make genuine attempts to rid himself of the influence of the traumatized self- and object-images that had been deposited in him by his stepfather. As he did so, he stopped being a malignant hunter and actually became an effective environmentalist. During the termination phase of his analysis, however, Peter was very much aware that if he ceased to be a reservoir for his stepfather's externalization, he might destabilize the older man's physical health. Such a prospect posed a major dilemma for Peter, but in the end he chose to get well as completely as possible. He eventually dismantled his trophy room and transformed it into a greenhouse where he worked with his wife, with whom he could now have a better relationship. He kept his job in the military-industrial complex, because it was the only work that he knew how to do well to earn a decent living, but his emotional involvement in missiles, guns, and other weapons of war faded away.

As Peter worked through his problems and prepared to finish his analysis, the stepfather, now in his 70s, seemed to sense that his decades-long externalizations were no longer stable. Because Peter was no longer an appropriate reservoir for his stepfather's externalized images and their associated affects, the old man's investment in the birdhouse, the other object of his externalized images, was also weakened. He laboriously uprooted the purple martin "apartment building," sold his house, and moved to a different state, leaving the birdhouse behind. Within days, he became seriously ill and suicidal; when he regained his strength, he decided to return to the original location where he had lived with Peter's mother. In order to do so, he made an offer to buy back his old house at nearly twice the price for which he had just sold it, but the new owner would not sell it back to him. Frustrated, he bought the house next door and became preoccupied with recreating the birdhouse. But the magic was gone; he never fully recovered. The hitherto successfully externalized traumatized images had returned to the self-representation of the individual who had externalized them in the first place.

The example of Peter's stepfather may help us elucidate how certain individuals, after a severely traumatic personal experience, are able to achieve a seemingly durable and asymptomatic adaptation. He was able to secure a precarious but functional "truce" with his externalizations instead of *working through* the underlying conflicts. In a sense, he was like the Jewish Holocaust survivor movingly described by Ira Brenner (1999a), who seemed to live a "normal" life in the United States because he had given to his children, unconsciously, various tasks that he himself wished to accomplish. Although we are not yet in a position to generalize because we have not accumulated sufficient clinical experience with such patients, the case of Peter's stepfather seems to suggest that traumatized self-images and associated internalized object-images may never disappear, even though some of them are absorbed in identifications. What we can say with certainty is that through their stable externalization individuals can free themselves from the pathological influences of their bruised parts. Such externalizations, however, are not without risks. There is always the danger that under certain circumstances—even decades later—the externalizations may "boomerang," returning to the original victim with dire consequences, as we observed with Peter's stepfather.

It is significant that one of Peter's children, a daughter, became a veterinarian; we can understand this career choice as an effort to repair the animals hurt by her father. Peter's case thus demonstrates the transgenerational transmission of a traumatized self-image and associated internalized object-images and affects across three generations of a family. It is important to note that as the traumatized images passed from one generation to another, the response changed; each generation assumed different tasks of displaced destruction, repair, and restoration, which they carried out unconsciously. We assume that the influence of what has been transmitted may become sublimated; we think that this was true for Peter's daughter. Nevertheless, we believe that transgenerational transmissions of this kind only cease when persons into whom traumatized images with associated affects have been deposited acquire insight into the influence of these on their mental life and behavior and are thus able to work through and to remove those influences from their self-representations.

Identification Versus Deposited Representation

It is especially clinical observations of transgenerational transmissions of self- or object-images like these three that point us toward the mechanism by which transgenerational transmission of historical trauma occurs. Can the transgenerational transmission of a raped-woman image or an imprisoned-man image be fully explained by the children's identifications with those images in the adults? We believe that identification alone cannot adequately explain this type of transgenerational transmission or that of second (and subsequent) generation(s) of a massively traumatized large group.

The common concept of *identification*, with which all clinicians will be familiar, refers to a subject's unconscious introjection and assimilation of another person's self-images—and the ego functions associated with them—through interactions with that other person. The processes of introjection and identification are usually accompanied by incorporative fantasies, such as imagining eating the object. True identification is only possible after children separate their self-representations from the representations of others. Under such conditions, what comes from outside modifies, to some degree, the child's self-representation. In the identification process, the child (or later the adult) is the active partner in the interaction.

By contrast, the concept of *deposited representation* (Volkan, 1987) emphasizes the role of the objects who unconsciously—and sometimes even consciously—force aspects of themselves, or aspects of their own internalized object-images, into the self-representations of children. By depositing images and representations into the child's developing (or a regressed adult's) self-representation, the object influences the child's sense of identity and gives the child certain specific tasks to perform. In fact, we have observed that other people can pass their images, with associated affects, to children even before children achieve an intrapsychic separation between their own psychic boundaries and those that belong to the object. In the process of deposited representation, the active partner is the other person, not the child (or regressed adult) whose self-representation functions as a reservoir. As psychoanalysts, we believe that Judith Kestenberg (1982) observed this depositing mechanism in action, in what she called the *transgenerational transportation* of trauma in the minds of Holocaust survivors who could not mourn losing objects murdered by the Nazis. The "deposited image" (Volkan, 1987) becomes like a psychological "gene" that influences the child's identity and self-representation, initiating certain tasks that the child is obliged to perform—though, again, without the parent or other caregiver ever verbalizing the demand.

Consider, for instance, the situation of the "replacement child" (Cain and Cain, 1964; Green and Solnit, 1964; Legg and Sherick, 1976; Poznanski, 1972; Volkan and Ast, 1997). Parents have a mental representation of their deceased children. When a second child is born after the death of the first, the child, of course, has no actual experience with the dead sibling. In relating to the second child, however, the parent actively requires the new child to interact with the mental representation of the deceased child that is carried internally. Sometimes, parents may even be partly conscious of what they are doing, naming the second child after the first or consciously noticing in the second child certain physical or personality aspects of the deceased one. In this sense, then, we say it is the parents who "deposit" their own internalized object-representation into the developing self-representation of the second child, a process that may start even before the child's symbiotic phase is over. Conveyed by interactions with the parent, this foreign psychological "gene" influences or modifies the replacement child's core identity. At the same time, the psychological gene manifests itself in tasks that the child is unconsciously impelled to perform: The child may feel obliged to repair the lost object so that the parent will be spared a complicated mourning and will therefore regain psychological health.

The case of Linda (Volkan, 1981) demonstrates how a replacement child may "experience [herself] as a depository of a representation of someone else as it existed in the minds of [her] parents" (Volkan, 1987, pp. 42–43). Linda's father was involved in complicated mourning over the death of his son, who died at 7 years of age. Linda, the daughter of a subsequent marriage, developed a mission to make her father forget his grief; she kept within herself her father's representation of the dead boy, whom she had never seen, and identified with it to a considerable extent, behaving on many occasions as if she were a boy. When she herself had a son, who now became the third generation affected by the trauma, she perceived him, at least for a while, as representative of her father's dead son, which, in turn, reactivated and complicated her oedipal fantasies.

Many survivors of a shared massive traumatic event are active in creating the dynamics of the replacement child, sometimes even consciously aware that their children symbolically replace relatives lost in the event. Again, the child is the recipient of an image belonging to the older person; now, however, that image is not of another child, but of a survivor's self- or object-image that is linked to historical trauma. Because the survivors have not resolved their conflicts about these images, it is they who initiate the passing of those images to the children, together with associated psychological tasks such as repairing the deposited images and reversing the humiliation of the events. The children, in turn, sense the survivors' pleasure or displeasure because of the survivors' reactions to this attempted transmission and may actively come to support the survivors' attempts to make the children reservoirs for this deposited image.

The next chapter explores how transgenerationally transmitted self- and object-images properly belonging to the survivors of massive shared trauma often initiate specifically history-related *unconscious fantasies* in their descendants, whose task it becomes to deal with the shame, rage, helplessness, entitlement, and guilt that the previous generation/s have been unable to work through for themselves.

4

History-Related
UNCONSCIOUS FANTASIES

As David Beres (1962) long ago noted, psychoanalysts detect the presence of unconscious fantasies only indirectly—that is, from their effects. Through listening to free associations, dreams, stories involving transference, and projective psychological tests, clinicians can discern the derivatives of such fantasies and, in time, put them into words. Once the "storyline" of an unconscious fantasy becomes conscious through therapeutic work, it closely resembles a conscious fantasy or daydream. Still, this storyline expresses primary process—which is to say, illogical—thinking. For example, a patient's previously unconscious fantasy, now verbalized, reads something like this: "I want to enter my mother's belly and kill my unborn sibling." As long as the fantasy remained unconscious, the psychoanalyst or therapist could only see its influence on the patient's dreams and symptoms; the patient might have suffered from claustrophobia, for instance, the enclosed spaces representing the mother's belly. Symptomatically, then, the patient avoids entering such spaces, but from a psychological point of view what she avoids is the sibling, made dangerous in the patient's mind by projections of her own childhood aggression or murderous rage onto the unborn fetus inside her mother's abdomen. Before her fantasy is made conscious, this patient may also have reported dreams reflecting similar themes, and these themes will have repeated themselves in the transference neurosis. (See Volkan and Ast, 1997, for many detailed examples of womb and sibling unconscious fantasies among more than a dozen of their patients.) The storyline of an unconscious fantasy—like a daydream—satisfies aggressive or sexual tensions, restores self-esteem, seeks satisfaction for various wishes, supports rebellion against or submission to superego or superego precursors, or performs any combination of these tasks. Once the fantasy is made conscious and is reflected in the transference neurosis, it can be worked through with the help of the analyst or therapist.

Freud (1908) noted two types of unconscious fantasy: those that "have been unconscious all along and have been formed in the unconscious; or—as is more often the case—[those that] were once conscious phantasies, day-dreams, and have since been purposely forgotten and have become unconscious through 're-pression'" (p. 161). Our focus here is not on the first type of unconscious fantasy, considered (especially by followers of Melanie Klein) to be a bridge between instinctual drives and thought; Kleinians would speak, for example, of the storyline of individuals' wish to attack their mothers' breasts as a derivative of the aggressive drive of nursing infants. Rather, our interest centers on the second type of unconscious fantasy Freud noted, which organizes drive derivatives by the child's experiences, especially traumatic ones. For a child's perception and "interpretation" of a childhood trauma to initiate an unconscious fantasy of the second type, it has to be repressed and to be influenced and distorted by primary process thinking. When this process occurs, it exerts, as unconscious "content," an interminable psychodynamic effect on subsequent perception, behavior, thinking, responses to reality, and other adaptive or maladaptive compromise formations (Arlow, 1969; Inderbitzin and Levy, 1990; Volkan and Ast, 1997).

We are extending the study of unconscious fantasies by positing that there exist unconscious (repressed) fantasies that are due neither to children's own traumatic experiences and their "interpretations" of those traumas, nor simply to the parents' own unconscious fantasies transmitted directly to children (such as the one that Carlos/Carla's mother had about her daughter having or being a penis, as described in chapter 3). Rather, we argue, there is another type of unconscious fantasy that is developed *solely* by the child from images of the traumatic experiences suffered by the large group or groups to which the child belongs; the shared mental representation of the group's history becomes connected to some aspect of the child's developmental conflicts and thus comes to appear in the "content" of such unconscious fantasies. "Because my arm is deformed and I am subject to extermination as a handicapped person under the Nazi regime, I need to create a symbolic repaired arm in order not to be exterminated." "I am a Nazi, and if I express my anger, I will destroy in a most sadistic manner the lives of those who have frustrated me; in order to keep this a secret, I need to smile all the time." "My abusive Jewish mother is Hitler and treats me like a Jew in a concentration camp." "I believe that my father was an SS officer, and the fact that he is my love-object has to be hidden, so I should repeat acts to deny my Germanness." Such storylines as these can profoundly influence all kinds of developmental processes and more typical unconscious fantasies—such as those pertaining to body functions, separation-individuation, the oedipus conflict, family romance, primal scenes, and sibling rivalry—and may be condensed with or coexist with parental fantasies transferred to children or children's own fantasies pertaining to their ancestors' actual individual traumas (and defenses against these).

What is new in our formulation is that this type of history-related unconscious fantasy does not stem from children's perceptions and "interpretations" of their own developmental traumas, conflicts, or both, but from children's reactions to images of their traumatized parents/ancestors *and* images of the general historical trauma their parents' group suffered that have been deposited in children by significant adults in the children's lives. In other words, the sources for such fantasies are not restricted to parents/ancestors' specific personal experiences. It is true that such children receive images, affects, and fantasies associated with their ancestors' actual individual experiences of trauma. But survivors of devastating trauma develop a sense of "belongingness" as a result of sharing the trauma, regardless of the fact that each person's trauma may be different, and despite the fact that most members of the group will never know or even meet one another. Common mental representations of their shared history become a kind of adhesive for their shared identity. In turn, the self- and object-images that survivors deposit into their offspring incorporate what derives from their new sense of interconnection: the shared representation of the collective history. As growing children accrue a fragmentary but more general knowledge of their group's historical suffering, then, they connect these other narratives of the group's trauma with the traumatized self- and object- (victim and victimizer) images that have been deposited in them by significant adults, at once reinforcing those deposited images and broadening the range of material for history-related fantasy. Regardless of the ancestors' personal experiences, then, the mental images of this history become inextricably intertwined with the individual child's developmental object relations and psychosexual conflicts. Thus a patient of nomadic heritage whose mother was not actually sterilized under the Third Reich—as were so many Gypsies—may nevertheless experience a Nazi-related unconscious fantasy that, once conscious, reads something like "Because I have Gypsy blood and therefore I am sterilized, I can have sex without fear of pregnancy." Parents, other significant adults, or both, impose and reinforce tasks of repair and restoration by relating to the child as a victim, a victimizer, or both—by relating to the self- and other-images of which they have made that child the carrier. Children develop *general* history-related unconscious fantasies because the traumatized self- and object-images passed on to children by their ancestors become amalgamated with their identity as a member of the traumatized large group, which is part of their core identity. Indeed, such unconscious fantasies actually serve to strengthen the bonds among those who share that large-group identification; this is the genesis of a *chosen trauma*.

Large Groups' Shared Chosen Tramua

Understanding "chosen trauma"—the mental representation of an event that has caused a large group to face drastic losses, to feel helpless and victimized by another group, and to share a humiliating injury—is key to discerning the process of transgenerational transmission of past historical events (Volkan, 1991a, 1992, 1997b, 1999a; Volkan and Itzkowitz, 1994). Although some have taken exception to the term *chosen* trauma because a group does not consciously choose to be victimized or suffer humiliation, we believe that, like an individual, a large group can be said to make unconscious "choices." Thus the term *chosen trauma* accurately reflects a large group's *unconscious* "choice" to add a past generation's mental representation of a shared event to its own identity. Although large groups may have experienced any number of traumas in their history, only certain ones remain alive over many years—indeed, often over a period of centuries. The chosen trauma forms thousands and millions of people designated—"chosen"—to be linked together through their shared mental representation of that trauma. A chosen trauma reflects the traumatized past generation's incapacity for or difficulty with mourning losses connected to the shared traumatic event, as well as its failure to reverse the humiliation and injury to the group's self-esteem ("narcissistic injury") inflicted by another large group, usually a geographical neighbor.

Although transgenerational transmission of large-group chosen trauma could plausibly be explained as a variation of such well-known psychological mechanisms as externalization, displacement, and identification, we believe it is sufficiently distinct from these mechanisms to be anatomized in its own right. When Peter's stepfather externalized his traumatized images with associated affects onto Peter, he externalized aspects of his own personal traumatic history, rather than that of the large group of which he was a member. That is, the Bataan Death March, though a horrific event for those who experienced it, never became a truly defining marker for the American people as a whole. Therefore, despite the fact that his psychopathology was formed in part by the world-historical experience of one of his caregivers, Peter's case cannot, properly speaking, be called a transgenerational transmission of large-group chosen trauma. When, however, a mental representation of massive collective trauma becomes an ethnic or national marker, it must become intertwined with the *core identity* of every (or almost every) individual member of the large group: this is what we call chosen trauma.

By "core identity" we refer to the individual's persistent and subjective sense of inner sameness (Erikson, 1956), which includes realistic body image, as well as "consistent attitudes, temporality, gender, authenticity, and ethnicity" (Akhtar and Samuel, 1996, p. 254). Revising Erikson's (1956) claim that "identity formation . . . begins where the usefulness of identification ends" (p. 113), Volkan (1997b) argues that "it is more accurate to say that formation of identity begins when the integration of early identifications is solidified" (p. 88). What differentiates people's core identity—which includes their large-group identity—from noncore (e.g., professional: "I am a photographer," etc.; or political: "I am a Democrat," etc.) subidentities is the degree of anxiety that individuals experience when they perceive danger to their psychic existence. Dissolution of one's core identity creates an overwhelming psychic shock and terror, as Ping-Nie Pao (1979) and Volkan (1995) observe in other contexts; when people decompensate into schizophrenia, for example, developing delusional identities (e.g., Jesus Christ, Mother Teresa) immediately following the shock phase, this represents the individuals' developmentally "primitive" attempts to escape the terror of losing their core identity. Threats to one's subidentities, on the other hand, do not produce anxiety of this magnitude. For example, individuals who have a subidentity as a photographer can change their profession and become carpenters without experiencing terror. If photographers changing professions experience anxiety over and above that warranted by realistically anxiety-producing factors (such as loss of income), the loss of their subidentity has become symbolic of one or another of the childhood calamities described by Freud (1926) as potential internal danger signals: the loss of the mother; the loss of the mother's love; the loss of a body part, or castration; and the loss of self-esteem, or failure to live up the expectations of one's ego-ideal and superego demands.

There is far more to transgenerational transmission of chosen trauma than children mimicking the behavior of parents or hearing stories of the event told by the older generation; nor is it a matter merely of transgenerational sympathy, powerful as that emotion may be. Rather, it is the end result of mostly unconscious psychological processes by which children's core identities are flooded with and therefore influenced by the injured self- and internalized object-images and associated affects that rightfully belong to the original victims, their caregivers or parents. As we have described, the representation of the drastic event is an integral part of all such deposited images, "piggybacking," so to speak, on the traumatized self- and object-images of the first-generation victim; no transmission of the event's representation can take place unless it is coupled with deposited self- and object-images and associated affects, because these are the only elements by which representations can be passed from a person of one generation to a person of another by assigning duties—specific tasks of reparation, reversal of helplessness, and so forth—to the next generation, mostly unconsciously. Thus people do not transmit to their progeny their memories of historical experience, for memory can belong only to the survivor of trauma and cannot be transmitted; survivors can only transmit aspects of themselves that contain a representation of history. It is for this reason that the effects of chosen trauma are so profound; the representation of history in the chosen trauma is intimately bound up with the very foundations of each group member's identity as an individual human being.

As injured self- and internalized object-images pass from generation to generation, the chosen trauma they carry assumes new functions, new tasks. The historical truth about the event is no longer of psychological moment for the large group; what is important is the sense of being linked together by the shared chosen trauma, which usually becomes highly mythologized. We believe, for example, that the forced exile, later return, and continuing anxiety of Kosovar

Albanians—who were forced to leave their homes by Serbian forces, who survived while others died, whose faces appeared on millions of television screens during the summer of 1999—will likely evolve into a large-group chosen trauma. Though individuals in an acutely traumatized large group have their own unique core identities, subidentities, and personal reactions to trauma, all members share mental representations of the tragedies that have befallen the group. Kosovar survivors' injured self- and internalized object-images connected to mental representations of the shared massive trauma will be deposited into the developing self-representations of their children, as if these children will be able to mourn the loss or reverse the humiliation and repair the injured images. If these children cannot confront and work through what has been deposited in them, they, as adults, will in turn pass the mental representations of the event to still another generation. Eventually, the event may evolve as a chosen trauma, be incorporated into the core identities of future generations of Kosovar Albanians and become an integral part of Kosovar Albanian identity.

Chosen traumas are often ritualistically recalled at the anniversary of the original event, when the members of the large group share an especially strong sense of group cohesion and belongingness. Czechs, for example, commemorate the battle of Bila Hora in 1620, which led to their subjugation under the Hapsburg Empire for nearly 300 years; Scots keep alive the story of the battle of Culloden in 1746, the failure of Bonnie Prince Charlie to restore a Stuart to the British throne. The Dakota Indians of the United States recall the anniversary of their decimation at Wounded Knee in 1890, and Crimean Tatars define themselves by the collective suffering of their deportation from Crimea in 1944. Some chosen traumas are difficult to detect because they are not simply connected to a single, easily recognizable past historical event. For instance, during the first four years after Estonia regained its independence from the Soviet Union in 1991, there appeared a generalized anxiety that Estonians as an ethnic group would disappear. This anxiety, it turned out, was connected with a reactivation of Estonians' chosen trauma, which was not related to one specific event but to the fact that they had lived under the dominance of other groups—Swedes, Germans, Russians—for a millennium, except for a brief period of independence between 1918 and 1940. Because of their history of submission, Estonians shared variations on the unconscious fantasy that they would once more be swallowed up by another group, a fantasy that served to unite them during the first three or four years after regaining independence. One-third of the 1.5 million people now living in Estonia are Russians (Russian speakers), a fact that played a significant role in the development of the shared fantasy. Intellectually, most Estonians were aware that the Russians living in the country needed to be integrated into the general population. Nevertheless, soon after Estonia's independence, even the most intelligent Estonians feared that placing as few as 2 Russian children in a kindergarten class with 16 Estonian ones would result, in a few months, in all the children speaking Russian, instead of the other way around. A project carried out in Estonia by the Center for the Study of Mind and Human Interaction (CSMHI) of Charlottesville, Virginia (in collaboration with the Carter Center in Atlanta, Georgia), showed the Estonian fantasy to be just that: a fantasy. Integrating the kindergarten classroom without either Estonian or Russian children losing their large-group identities proved quite possible; indeed, the Estonian government is itself now expanding the original CSMHI project (Apprey, 1996; Apprey et al., 2000; Neu and Volkan, 1999; Volkan, 1997b). Because their identity as an occupied and oppressed group is no longer reflected in the nation's political reality, Estonians now have to rediscover a "new" group identity.

A chosen trauma may or may not be readily evident at all times; it may lie dormant for a long period of time, like unconscious conflicts in an individual that are effectively repressed; yet, like such individual conflicts, the chosen trauma can be reactivated to exert a powerful psychological force in the lives of the group members. Indeed, certain political leaders seem intuitively to know how to reactivate a chosen trauma, especially when their large group is in conflict or has gone through a radical change and needs to reconfirm or enhance its identity. Chosen trauma acts like a fuel to maintain large-group conflicts, even if the conflicts have their origins in economic, legal, political, or military controversy.

Time Collapse

Time collapse is the term we use to denote the conscious and unconscious connections between past trauma and present threat that typically emerge when a chosen trauma is powerfully reactivated. Rekindling shared anxieties, expectations, fantasies, and defenses associated with the chosen trauma naturally magnifies the image of current enemies and current conflicts. If the large group is now in a powerful position, the sense of revenge may become exaggerated, even ennobled. If the large group is in a powerless position, a current event may reanimate a shared sense of victimization. Time collapse may lead to irrational and sadistic or masochistic decision-making by the leadership of the large group; in turn, members of the large group may become psychologically prepared for sadistic or masochistic acts, and, in the worst-case scenario, may perpetrate otherwise unimaginably monstrous cruelty against others. The conscious and unconscious aim of such decisions and acts is to protect the group's shared identity (Volkan et al., 1998). The history of ethnic Serbs in the late 1980s and 1990s provides a prime example of such time-collapsed chosen trauma reactivation.

After becoming independent from Byzantium in the 12th century, the Kingdom of Serbia thrived for almost 200 years under the leadership of the Nemanjić dynasty, reaching its zenith under the beloved Emperor Stefan Dušan. After Dušan died in 1355, the Nemanjić dynasty soon came to an end. In 1371, Serb feudal lords elected Lazar Hrebeljanović as leader of Serbia, although he assumed the title of prince rather than tzar. The decline of Serbia that followed his ascension to power is primarily attributed to the expansion of the Ottoman Empire into Serb territory, culminating in the Battle of Kosovo on June 28, 1389, at the *Kosovo Polje* ("Field of the Black Birds"). Though there are various versions of the "historical truth" of the Battle of Kosovo (Emmert, 1990), it is certain that the leaders of both warring groups were killed and that Lazar's body was canonized and mummified. Later, the mummified remains of Lazar were moved from a monastery near the battleground to a safer location north of Belgrade, as the Ottomans consolidated their control over Serb territory. During this same period, the Battle of Kosovo, which had begun earlier to evolve into a chosen trauma for the Serb people, truly crystallized into a most important ethnic marker. Mythologized tales of the battle and Prince Lazar were passed from generation to generation through the strong Serbian oral and religious tradition, perpetuating and reinforcing Serbs' traumatized self-images (Emmert, 1990; Lazarovich-Hrebelianovich and Calhoun, 1910; Markovic, 1983; Volkan, 1997b, 1999a).

In April 1987, as the 600th anniversary of the Battle of Kosovo approached, Slobodan Milošević, former president of present-day Yugoslavia (the Serb-Montenegro federation) and then a Communist bureaucrat, was attending a meeting of 300 party delegates in Kosovo. At the time, only 10 percent of the population in Kosovo was Serbian; the majority consisted of Albanian Muslims. During the meeting, a crowd of Serbs and Montenegrins tried to force its way into the meeting hall. Its members wanted to voice grievances about the hardships they were experiencing in Kosovo, but the local police blocked and prohibited their entrance into the meeting hall. At that moment, Milošević stepped forward and exclaimed: "Nobody, either now or in the future, has the right to beat you." Enraptured by the drama of the moment, the crowd became frenzied and spontaneously began to sing "Hej Sloveni," the national anthem, and shouted, "We want freedom! We will not give up Kosovo!" This response in turn excited Milošević; he remained in the building until dawn—a 13-hour period—to listen to tales of Serb victimization at the hands of Kosovo Muslims. Milošević emerged from this experience a transformed leader, clad in the armor of Serb nationalism. He would later declare in a speech that Serbs in Kosovo are not a minority because "Kosovo is Serbia and will always be Serbia."

One action in particular exemplifies how Milošević, with the help of some academics and the Serbian Church, reactivated the Serbian chosen trauma and re-empowered Serb nationalism. In 1889, the 500th anniversary of Kosovo, plans for moving Prince Lazar's mummified body back to the Kosovo region had been discussed, but never came to fruition. As the 600th anniversary neared, Milošević, together with others in his political circle, and with the blessing of the Serbian Orthodox Church, decided to bring Lazar's body "out of exile." Soon thereafter, the mummified remains of the legendary leader of the Serbs were placed in a coffin and taken "on tour" to every Serb village and town, where the body was met by throngs of mourners dressed in black, along with church leaders clad in religious garb. Serbs began to feel the effects of the collapse of 600 years into the present. As they greeted Lazar's body, they cried and wailed and solemnly vowed in speeches never to allow such a defeat to occur again. The "tour" of Lazar's body functioned, in essence, as a daily reincarnation and reburial of the medieval prince.

In reactivating Serbs' mental image of Lazar, Milošević apparently made space for the group to grieve Lazar's (and its) defeat at the Battle of Kosovo at last. Instead of focusing on grief, however, the Serbian propaganda machinery emphasized the need to reverse the unacceptable feelings of helplessness, humiliation, and shame. Mourners appeared to feel afresh affects appropriate to traumatized self-images, bonding the modern-day Serbs more closely together; individual Serbs' self-images became suffused with a new sense of common entitlement for revenge. It is unclear whether Milošević *intended* to generate this response; whether intentional or not, however, the reactivation of the Serbs' chosen trauma clearly played a significant role in creating the atmosphere in which atrocities against Bosniaks (Bosnian Muslims), and later against Kosovar Albanians (also Muslims), could take place, since Serbs have historically perceived both Bosniaks and Albanians as extensions of the Ottomans. (For a more detailed account of the Serbs' chosen trauma and its reactivation, see Volkan, 1997b, 1999a.)

Jews around the globe, including those not personally affected by the Holocaust, all to some degree define their large-group identity by direct or indirect reference to the Holocaust. The shared mental representation of the Holocaust has evolved as a significant ethnic marker, even though Orthodox Jews still refer to the 586 B.C.E. destruction of the Jewish temple in Jerusalem by Nebuchadnezzar II of Babylonia as *the* chosen trauma of the Jews, and despite the fact that Israelis of Middle Eastern and African origin sometimes report that they are less affected by the Holocaust than are other Jews. In order for the Holocaust to crystallize fully into a chosen trauma as we have described it here, however, decades of further transgenerational transmission will be required.

We have gathered in this book the cases of a number of second-generation Holocaust victims who have come to us for treatment. Our case reports emphasize not large-group psychology or the psychology of the chosen trauma, but rather the transgenerational transmission of still relatively "hot" trauma. By examining their inner worlds, we can discern in minute detail what takes place in the initial stages of chosen trauma evolution. By tracking how general history-related unconscious fantasies coexist with other transgenerational transmissions, our detailed case studies illuminate how the offspring of a victimized generation are drawn together in closer identification with one another, influencing the core individual and large-group identities of generations to come.

Part 2
CASE STUDIES

5

Jacob

THE INABILITY TO MOURN

A JEWISH MAN WHO SPENT THE FIRST 17 MONTHS of his life in hiding in Nazi-occupied Belgium, Jacob first entered therapy at the age of 27, when he was hospitalized after a suicide attempt. During Jacob's treatment with a young psychiatrist under Dr. Volkan's supervision, it became clear that Jacob was in a state of complicated mourning for his Holocaust survivor father, who had died when Jacob was 12. Like the two young men described by Freud (1927) who had lost their fathers as children, Jacob used splitting and vacillated between two assumptions: "one being that his father was still alive and was hindering him from action, and the other being that his father was dead which gave him the right to regard himself as his successor" (p. 156). While we recognize that there were additional personal reasons that contributed to Jacob's extreme difficulties, these personal elements were typical of what is familiar from other clinical work with complicated mourners. What is most interesting here is the role of the Holocaust's legacy in Jacob's perennial mourning. As we eventually learned, the matrix of Jacob's self-representation was saturated with the Nazi period to such an extent that it could not allow him to grieve his father's death.

Jacob's Personal History

Jacob's life began most unusually. Just before his birth, his mother emerged from hiding by avowing that she was not Jewish. By accepting the false status of illegitimacy for her child even though she and Jacob's father had in fact been lawfully married, she was thus able to give birth to Jacob in a hospital. There, she was able to ask Jews employed in the hospital to circumcise her son, a bold move by a Jewish woman determined to cling to a Jewish identity for herself and her child in the face of grave danger. After this daring delivery, she rejoined her husband and another Jewish couple with a small daughter in hiding. They remained there for another 17 months, with the new baby sleeping in a dresser-drawer.

Though the family left its hiding place as soon as Belgium was liberated, family members remained in the country, where the father worked as a tailor, for five years. Soon after liberation, Jacob's father began to have multiple, recurrent somatic symptoms. When Jacob was about 7, the family members moved to New York and became naturalized citizens of the United States. There, his father started a tailoring business, which became rather successful. He soon became frustrated, however, and constantly complained at the most minor irritants. Based on Jacob's account of his father, it would seem that the father had developed many of the symptoms of a classic case of survivor syndrome, as described by William Niederland (1968; see also chapter 1). Suffering from sleep disturbance, phobias, and depressed states, he withdrew into an angry, morose, and brooding state of isolation. Furthermore, he showed resomatization of affect (Hoppe, 1968; Schur, 1955), suffering a peptic ulcer. Although Jacob's father had not undergone the harrowing experience of living in a concentration camp, he had nonetheless been in constant danger during his period in hiding, because the family that sheltered the fugitives was aiding them for mercenary, rather than compassionate, reasons. He had also been aware of what awaited him and his family if they were caught; before going into hiding in Belgium, Jacob's father had once been apprehended by the Nazis, but had escaped by jumping off a train. Having left Poland before the Nazi invasion, Jacob's parents presumed that relatives left behind had fallen victim to the Nazis.

When Jacob was about 12, his father was diagnosed with multiple sclerosis, which progressed very rapidly: After a year of increasing disability, during which Jacob bore considerable responsibility for the man's bodily care, he died. On the surface, Jacob appeared to deal with his father's death as well as could be expected for a boy his age; despite not being able to speak English when he came to the United States, he continued to earn good grades in school after his father's death. His mother did not remarry, but continued to work in the tailor shop. Shortly after her husband's death, she appeared on a television show to tell of her family's ordeal and to appeal for sympathy and financial aid, and she encouraged Jacob to seek help also. He got free food at the school cafeteria for his efforts, but felt that his mother had made a supplicant of him. Though he complained bitterly, he adhered to this role in years to come and always felt dissatisfied. Nevertheless, he graduated from college, where he was an average student. After marrying a Jewish woman whom he perceived to be a Zionist, he moved with his wife to the city in which Dr. Volkan practices, in order to pursue postgraduate studies.

Jacob first came to Dr. Volkan's attention after an abortive suicide attempt with sleeping pills, shortly after a week-long visit from his mother. It became evident later that his acute and overt depression had been precipitated by her visit, which had brought him to a sudden conscious realization that both of them were living in what he called "emotional prisons." As Jacob saw it, his mother was "imprisoned" by continuing to live in the old neighborhood in New York, even though it was deteriorating; she had twice been harassed by the hoodlums who now inhabited the area. When she refused his pleas to move out of the neighborhood, Jacob realized that, like her, he was also living in a "prison." He was not enjoying his wife, his graduate school classmates or neighbors, or life in general.

Mourning and the Holocaust

Before detailing Jacob's case, we should ask why so many Holocaust survivors and their offspring develop complicated mourning reactions to their losses—that is, either an inability to mourn or difficulty in mourning. To answer this question, it is necessary to review the nature of "normal" mourning, the obligatory adult human reaction to loss or threat of loss.

Psychoanalysts have long disagreed on the question of when a child is capable of mourning. Those who subscribe to John Bowlby's (1960, 1969) "attachment theory" claim that mourning is possible in infancy, but many psychoanalysts agree with Anna Freud's (1960) view that prior to the development of *object constancy*—that is, prior to the time that the image of a cathected person can be maintained internally, irrespective of frustration or satisfaction—the pleasure-pain principle governs the child's response to a loss. We agree with those colleagues who hold that the child's internal process of mourning prior to the full development of object constancy differs from that of adults; in fact, in our view, the individual must have successfully negotiated the adolescent passage truly to mourn like an adult (Wolfenstein, 1966, 1969).

The literature on mourning offers many taxonomies of the process, varying substantially on the investigators' phenomenological preferences. Following Volkan (Volkan, 1981; Volkan and Zintl, 1993), we focus on the mourner's internal processes after a loss, and, like George Pollock (1989), divide the mourning process into two steps: the *initial stage* and the *work of mourning.*

Adult mourning following the death of a loved one illustrates these two stages clearly. The *initial stage* includes the phase of numbness and shock; denial of death, followed by the splitting of ego functions (Freud, 1940) regarding the perception of death; the activation of certain images of the deceased and of inner relatedness to them; painful emotions accompanied by weeping; and the appearance of anger, indicating the ego's attempt to accept the loss and its psychological implications. This anger initiates the integration of the previously split ego functions in service to the reality principle—meaning that the emotional acceptance of death has begun. If no complications interpose, manifestations of the initial stage will disappear within 2 to 6 months after the death, depending on the circumstances of its occurrence and the mourner's own existing psychic organization. During this period, signs of the initial stage do not necessarily follow one another in strict order, but may suddenly disappear and re-appear again; mourners suffer because they search repeatedly for the lost object and are frustrated by not finding it.

As mourners' acceptance of the loss becomes more and more an internal process, the *work of mourning* begins in earnest, generally lasting for a year or so until mourners pass anniversaries of psychologically important events that they shared with the lost person. The work of mourning, as Freud (1917b) illustrated long ago, includes a "slow-motion," piecemeal review of the relationship to the deceased, as well as a struggle to keep or to reject a close internal tie with the deceased's various images. During this work, an initial regressive disorganization is followed by a new inner organization, a succession similar to that which occurs developmentally during the adolescent passage. With the development of this new inner organization, the mourner tests reality more fully for confirmation that the death, with all its psychological implications, has indeed taken place. The mourner now also becomes free to invest in new objects and their representations.

When the process of mourning is "normal," the mourner necessarily identifies adaptively and selectively with the lost person's images and with functions that are attached to those images. These selective identifications with images of the lost person enrich the mourner's internal world. Furthermore, when the normal course of mourning is as nearly complete as it ever becomes, the representation of the lost object becomes a "remembrance formation" (Tähkä, 1984), and the mourner views the lost object as a memory without a future: its representation can no longer provide the expected gratification for the mourner's libidinal or aggressive demands, conscious or unconscious.

Many factors, external and internal, may "infect" either the initial stage or the work of mourning, causing complications that can range from mild to severe—at the most severe, inability to mourn. Sudden death, for instance, usually creates difficulties. Stephen Shanfield and his colleagues (1986–87) found that parents who had lost adult children in sudden, traumatic ways, such as traffic accidents, developed significantly more problems in mourning than parents who lost children to chronic illnesses such as cancer. On the other hand, internal factors such as unresolved past losses and a psychic organization that makes the mourner dependent on others and intolerant of separations (Fenichel, 1945), may also create problems in the initial stage of mourning, the work of mourning, or both. We hold that the victims of a horror such as the Holocaust will *necessarily* have severe complications in their mourning processes and are more likely to experience the inability to mourn. As discussed previously, mourning is accompanied by anger, which connotes the ego's acceptance of the reality of the loss and thereby allows the mourning process to continue on from the initial stage. Victims of such massive horrors cannot experience this "normal" anger because of their feelings of guilt; in their unconscious and even conscious experience, anger actually kills others. Comparing unresolved grief to the survivor syndrome, William Niederland (1968) suggests that rage and resentment against the dead underlie the self-reproaches of those who survived the Holocaust, and that mourning is impossible for survivors because they feel the need to escape from the guilt that such resentment evokes in them.

Although we concur with Niederland, we would add several additional observations. First, we see survivors attempting, to a considerable extent, to deny their libidinal attachment to those they have lost, since doing so would induce guilt for not having been able to protect those people. The work of mourning requires an incremental review of both libidinal and aggressive experiences with those who are lost, but survivor guilt militates against this retrospection. Second, overt expressions of emotion and processes of rebelling and bargaining are not possible for those who have internalized a sense of helplessness against persecution and the need to remain silent at the peril of their lives. Indeed, this situation in itself would be sufficient to create difficulties in mourning or an inability to mourn. Third, massively horrific events induce an incredible state of helpless dependence that obliges victims to cling to external objects and their external representations, even when these objects or representations are actually dangerous—for example, when they are representations of the persecutors. This clinging is hidden behind a denial of attachment to the external object and its representation, as explained earlier. If they do not clutch the external object, the helpless and dependent victims unconsciously expect psychological annihilation. But as long as the victim clings in order to survive physically and psychically, the process of mourning—which aims to surrender the individual's investment in an object and its representation—cannot progress, and remembrance formations cannot be established. The victim cannot abandon the mental images or total representation of lost objects under these circumstances because of their vital role in maintaining psychic cohesion—as implied by Paul Chodoff's (1970) observation that survivors are extremely sensitive to actual or threatened separation from those upon whom they have become dependent.

Fourth, Holocaust survivors cannot achieve a remembrance formation and, therefore, cannot fully mourn. The feelings, perceptions, thoughts, and meanings connected with representations of the lost object or objects are, to us, the most important factors in the inability to mourn or extreme difficulty in mourning. In the Holocaust, the images of loss (of loved ones, self-esteem, community ties, physical possessions, and so on) were inconceivably great. The "memory" of the Holocaust cannot become integrated with other memories of a victim's personal experiences because the affects and meanings contained in it are simply too immense to be made into remembrance formations. To complete the mourning process would require forgiving and forgetting, which would induce the unbearable anxiety that the horror, with its assault to the sense of self, might then recur. Rafael Moses' (1984) writings on the loss of security in Holocaust survivors' interpersonal worlds reflect the fact that for these victims, it seems better to cling to the "memory" and be perennially on guard.

Fifth, and finally, when a loss is too great to be mourned, the survivor forms a closer identification with others in the large group who have lived through similar experiences, collectively thwarting the mourning process; indeed, the large-group cohesion that must be maintained to survive a massive trauma essentially *demands* that no mourning take place. If survivors truly mourn their losses, they will be freed from the intense relationship with the lost objects' representations that characterizes melancholia and perennial mourning. But in achieving this disengagement, those individuals will also separate themselves from the others in the group who remain attached to those representations in the common state of complicated mourning. Thus endeavoring to mourn alone almost necessarily induces guilt and a sense of loneliness. Many observers have noted that survivors of the Holocaust who moved to a new location after the war—for example, New York City—clustered themselves in apartment blocks in order to avoid the threat of this loneliness, to share their identities as victims/survivors. Although some survivors are better adjusted than others, a survivor need not present an overtly pathological picture to have been affected, for the damage is intrapsychic. Since the surface picture depends on defensive and adaptive mechanisms, it sometimes requires close scrutiny to observe hidden psychodynamics of extreme difficulty in mourning or the inability to mourn.

In chapter 2, we stated that the outcome of the work of mourning depends on what the mourner does, in the long run, with the representation of the lost person or thing. If the end result is not the completion of a "normal" mourning, the mourner may develop depression (melancholia) by identifying totally with the representation of the lost object, fully contaminated with love, hate, guilt, and helplessness. This total identification transforms the mourner's self-representation into the site of a debilitating struggle to contain the ambivalence and conflicts associated with the representation of the lost object or thing. The object-representation, now part of the mourner's self-representation, psychologically conquers and ruins the previously uncontaminated area of the mourner's internal world; individuals who exhibit classic survivor syndrome suffer from such depressive conditions. Other survivors become perennial mourners: doomed to perform tasks related to the work of mourning over and over without resolution. Neither can the offspring of survivors with such complicated mourning reactions perform their own work of mourning following a loss. Because their parents have passed to them the task of performing an impossible work of mourning and have been unable to "teach" their children the ego functions necessary for "normal" mourning, the offspring of survivors tend themselves to become perennial mourners as well.

Perennial Mourning

Before we examine more closely the case of Jacob, a perennial mourner directly affected by the Third Reich, however, let us first look at perennial mourning more generally, as it appears as a response to routine life experiences. Perennial mourners keep alive an illusion of continuing communication with the deceased, communication over which mourners feel themselves in absolute control. In fact, this "communication" is an inner dialogue with the mental representation of the deceased. This mental representation exists in mourners' minds as an *introject*, a specific kind of object-representation that mourners strive, but fail, to assimilate into their self-representation in the form of an identification. Subjectively experienced as an inner presence within the mourner's mind or body, the mourner maintains a continuous contact with the lost object, which continues to exert an influence on the mourner's self-representation. Of course, the introject is not a faithful replica of the external object, but rather is shaped by the mourner's wishes, fantasies, affects, and defenses against them.

A patient we will call Ted provides a striking example of an introject. During his diagnostic interview, Ted spoke of having problems with his older brother, Randolph. On the way to work, and increasingly on the way home, Ted complained; Randolph lectured him. Ted found these advice-laden monologues stressful after a long day at the office. It was not until halfway into the session that Ted mentioned that Randolph had been killed several years earlier in a hunting accident and that he felt that Randolph's head was lodged in his chest (Volkan and Zintl, 1993).

Most perennial mourners, of course, do not give such clear evidence of the presence of an introject; instead, they are more prone to speak of their *linking objects* (Volkan, 1981)—metapsychologically speaking, externalized versions of introjects. Perennial mourners develop linking objects (or linking phenomena) to serve as a symbolic bridge to their mental representations of the deceased; condensed in these magical things are the mourners' mental images of the deceased and their corresponding mental images of themselves. For mourners, these objects become an external point of contact between these two images over which they exert absolute control. Through linking objects, perennial mourners think of themselves as able to restore the dead to life, or to "kill" their lost objects themselves. Thus the mourner attempts to recreate and then to resolve the ambivalence that characterized the relationship prior to the person's death: an attempt to initiate or complete the work of mourning that never completes itself.

Many examples of linking objects and phenomena appear in the psychoanalytic and psychological literature. Linking objects are distinctive because they are generally not used according to their own original purpose, except on special occasions such as anniversaries. For example, a dead mother's bracelet, which had become a linking object for her daughter, was kept locked in a drawer in the daughter's bedroom; the daughter only wore it on the anniversary of her mother's death. But mourners always know the linking object's whereabouts, even though they may simply ignore it for a period of time. When using the linking object, the mourner is under its spell. The mourner jealously protects the linking object to maintain the process of mourning–which, since it is externalized, is not worked through. A linking phenomenon serves the same psychological functions. For example, instead of mourning her father, who had shot himself through the head, one young woman would recall the song "Raindrops Keep Falling on My Head." This song connected the image of the dead father with a bullet hole in his head to the corresponding image of his "crying" daughter (raindrops) *externally*. Thus, the young woman's *internal* work of mourning remained frozen.

Dina Wardi (1992) describes a kind of linking object used by a Holocaust survivor whose daughter, Hanna, was Wardi's patient. On Passover, when everyone would get dressed for the Seder, this man would put on a striped shirt he had kept from Auschwitz. Of course, this man's family members could not help but observe the peculiar use of his linking object; Wardi believes that Hanna's father chose to use the linking object in such a public manner in order to transmit cognitive and emotional messages about the Holocaust quite concretely to his daughter. The legacy of such transgenerational transmissions is that offspring of Holocaust survivors themselves often experience the inability to mourn or difficulty in mourning. In the case of Jacob, a perennial mourner who, on occasion, temporarily exhibited acute depression, the inability to mourn (or, at least, extreme difficulty in mourning) his father's death was intertwined with his inability to confront the impact of what had happened to his family during the Holocaust.

Jacob's Perennial Mourning

When Jacob, married for one year and childless, entered treatment, he was aware, deep down, that he had not resolved the issue of his father's death. Intellectually, Jacob had long acknowledged his father's death, while, at the same time, keeping him emotionally "alive." When he was in his mid-teens, for instance, a few years after his father's death, he saw a man on the street who, from behind, resembled his father. In order "to be sure" that it was not his father returned from the dead, he felt compelled to run past the stranger, turn, and look him in the face. At college, he felt that one of his teachers closely resembled his father—at times, the likeness seemed so strong that it very nearly led Jacob to break with reality. Interestingly, this professor's name was "Croak," a word Jacob often used in the colloquial sense of "die."

Over the years, Jacob had made a number of unhealthy and nonadaptive attempts to identify with his father. At the time of his father's death, Jacob's mother had prevented her son from participating in the customary Jewish mourning rituals and had sent him away instead to a camp in the country for "fresh air." While in the country, preoccupied with the thought of his father's decaying dead body, he caught and killed a snake by submerging it in a bottle of acid. Watching in fascination as the snake disintegrated, Jacob was clearly attempting to "kill" his father. Instead of "killing" his representation of his father in the psychological realm as part of his mourning process, however, Jacob felt a need to reenact it symbolically in the external world; it was as if he needed to see the decaying flesh of the snake (a symbol for the father) in order to believe that a death had really occurred. This need to externalize reflects Jacob's difficulty in mourning. Interestingly, Jacob also developed boils at the time of the snake-killing episode. Although there were probably physiological causes for his skin disease, psychological triggering seems evident here as well. Jacob could not develop selective identification with the "good" elements of his father's representation; his disruptive identification (with ambivalence) quite literally made him ill.

Another maladaptive identification arose after Jacob was injured in a street fight at the age of 16. While in the hospital recovering from a ruptured spleen, he donned the robe his father had worn during his final illness and used a wheelchair, as his father had done. Instead of feeling comforted by wearing his father's robe, however, Jacob reported having felt anxiety. He temporarily realized the death wish for his father that he had developed when the older man was still alive, ill, and wearing the robe himself. At the same time, Jacob reported, he had clearly sensed the presence of his father within his chest; his father had become an introject. His desire to express aggression against his father's introject made him feel guilty.

Visiting his father's grave just before leaving home for college induced another anxious temporary internalization experience for Jacob. Having made only two visits since his father's burial, he seems to have preferred to deny the existence of the grave—and thus to deny his father's death. The first of his prior visits had been when the tombstone was placed, one year after his father's death; a disagreeable exchange had taken place between his mother and a distant relative at that time, but Jacob recalled having had no symptoms then. Years later, in his early 20s and on the verge of leaving for college, he felt that he must say goodbye to his father. At the gravesite, Jacob experienced a sense of merging with the man buried there, a feeling that he could enter the grave and be one with him.

Such *merging* (or *fusing*) *identifications* are different from those that follow a process of *introjecting* the object-image. Introjections are usually accompanied by overt or covert cannibalistic fantasies, ending with the assimilation of the introjected object-image to the individual's self-representation. It is generally a gradual process, and the resulting identification is solid; the individual who has identified selectively with the object-image in this way enriches his ego functions and can now perform the ego functions previously performed by the object. On the other hand, if mourners have identified totally (that is to say, with ambivalence) with the image of the lost person, their internal world will become a site of struggle between the wish to repair and regain the lost object and the wish to "kill" that person. On the other hand, the merging type of identification is quick and temporary, and the individual is aware of the fusion process. The perennial mourner—who ordinarily does not maintain a solid identification with the lost object's representation—can, on occasion, exhibit temporary merging identifications. These experiences can, of course, be fatal for perennial mourners if they attempt to actualize the fantasy of merging with the deceased; otherwise, perennial mourners are not prone to suicide—unlike people who develop depression following a loss, who want to "kill" their identification with the representation of the lost object. Developing an introject and especially a linking object generally protects perennial mourners from suicide, because they are able to control the wish to bring the deceased to life or to "kill" that person.

Jacob had also established a panoply of linking objects, all broken, all representing the broken father with a crippling illness and Jacob's own corresponding images; only two representative examples will be noted. The significance of his father's broken pocket watch lay totally in Jacob's unconscious and became clear to him only during treatment. The initials on the back of the watch were his father's, SM; reversed, they gave the common name for his father's disease. But the watch therefore served not only as a perfect representation of the man broken with multiple sclerosis ("MS"), but also as a reflection of Jacob's feared total identification with that man. Preparing for the crucial exam in his master's of science degree program had been another internal factor in Jacob's suicide attempt. It was as if, symbolically, earning the degree would mean developing the illness called by the same name as the degree; receiving the M.S. would result in a total identification with the dead father known as SM.

The second item was a camera, also broken, which had hung for many years in the closet where Jacob kept his clothes, so that he saw it every day while dressing. That there was something peculiar about his keeping this useless thing had not occurred to him. He had once taken it for repair, but had been told that it would be expensive to put the broken camera in working order. The broken camera represented his sick father, and he "loved" it; because he also "hated" it, however, he refused to have it repaired. It was, in a sense, "the skeleton in the closet."

The session in which Jacob told his therapist about the camera clearly illustrates its significance to his unconscious mind, though he was not conscious of its meaning. The camera had a syringe-like attachment called a "time delayer," but Jacob had trouble remembering its name, suggesting that he himself was trying to delay or postpone something. After recalling the name of the attachment, he wept and talked of the experience of grief. Jacob then recollected having given injections to his dying father and remembered the flaccid appearance of the man's flesh. He recalled having fantasized that when he helped his father to the toilet, the older man would be flushed away. Continuing to associate,

Jacob mentioned that the camera attachment also reminded him of a snake. This association recalled for Jacob how modest his father had been—how, even in his weakened condition, he had been careful to keep his son from seeing his penis. But, concluded Jacob, his father had been verbally harsh and had complained endlessly.

In life, Jacob and his father had engaged in a highly ambivalent relationship; his father had at times been brutal toward the boy in the pattern of other survivors of Nazi persecution observed by de Wind (1968). In treatment, Jacob reported many dreams that reflected this ambivalence. On one occasion, Jacob dreamed of being wrapped in chains in a room that shrank and collapsed around him. This dream at once reflected an identification with the representation of his father, who had been in an iron lung, as well as an association with the period of confinement in hiding. In the first part of another dream, he was negotiating his father's release from a concentration camp, becoming his father's savior; this part of the dream was motivated by a desire to have a parent who was "saved" or "repaired" so that he could help his son up the developmental ladder. In the second part of the same dream, however, Jacob pushed his father into a toilet, recalling the sickroom fantasies of flushing his father away. Together, the two parts of the dream dramatically illustrate the struggle between the wish to bring the image of the dead object to life and the wish to "kill" it. This second dream is, in fact, typical of perennial mourners, who often have recurrent dreams in which the deceased is alive, usually undisguised, and frequently engaged in a life-and-death struggle. Mourners usually report having attempted rescue in the dream—which they frequently describe as having a "frozen" quality (Volkan, 1981)—but awakening before the dream goes further. Indeed, Jacob had many such recurrent dreams of trying to save his father—nightmares from which he would awaken before the issue of whether he was going to save his father was resolved.

Jacob lost his father at age 12, early in the period of development through which, as was mentioned previously, successful passage constitutes the sine qua non for the ability to mourn later in life. Martha Wolfenstein (1966, 1969) has noted that the adolescent passage is indeed a kind of "natural" rehearsal for adult mourning, involving the same psychodynamics. During the adolescent passage, individuals internally review their childhood relationship to the mental representations of parents and other significant individuals and relax their emotional investment in these people in order to transfer allegiance to peers and to enlarge their world. During this period, the young person also selectively re-identifies or dis-identifies with object-images of the past. Jacob thus bore a double burden, not only having to face the death of his father while an adolescent, but also being an heir to survivor syndrome. The first circumstance hindered his developmental model of mourning, as well as his emotional maturation process more generally, and the second misfortune complicated his mourning process still further.

Jacob's Assimilation of the Third Reich Experience in Perennial Mourning

Though Jacob could not establish a solid selective identification with the representation of his dead father, he clearly identified with his persecuted parents. Like his father, he responded to stress with psychosomatic conditions such as stomach ailments, persistent nightmares, and recurrent depressive episodes. Furthermore, although Jacob had been an infant during his period in hiding, he reported certain "memories" as if he had been an adult at the time. He would say that he had owned a radio, or "My mother would salvage strings of spinach from garbage and make soup," or "Sometimes we needed a bath, but had no soap." He felt that he had lived through those dreadful times in Belgium as a conscious adult and spontaneously compared his saga to that of Anne Frank. To him, these anecdotes were "memories," although they had been derived secondhand from stories his parents had recounted again and again, because he was, we believe, a reservoir for his victimized parents' deposited images.

It was impossible for him to mourn normally by reviewing the meanings of the lost father's representation because Jacob's self-representation was already a stable reservoir for his father's (and his mother's) traumatized images—images of them as victims of the Third Reich. Reviewing his dead father's representation would have meant reviewing his own internal world, exposing himself to intolerable feelings of victimhood. Instead, Jacob tried to deny and to avoid, as much as he could, his internalized images connected with the Third Reich. He had done so all along, not only by avoiding his father's grave, but also by evading religious ceremonies and discussions of Nazi persecution. Fascinated by certain words—*Holocaust*, *Nazi*, and the like—he avoided reading anything concerning the persecution of Jews. His denial and avoidance did not help him to live functionally, though, and thus, Jacob, as the reservoir of his parents' traumatized images, remained a "doomed Jew." As a child learning English in the United States, he had special difficulty learning the word *exit*, in spite of the fact that signs bearing the word appeared everywhere. As an adult, he demonstrated "selective blindness" by not seeing the exit signs in cinemas. There had been no exit from their hiding place in Belgium; there had been no exit to freedom for a Jew under the Third Reich.

Paradoxical as it may seem, Jacob's overall identification with his survivor parents and function as a reservoir for their deposited images coexisted with periodic identification with the Nazis. As was mentioned previously, Jacob was sent away "to get fresh air" in a "camp" during the first week after his father's death. In treatment, Jacob understood that his mother had ambivalently wanted her child to be free and have fresh air—but, after all, had sent him to a "camp," which reminded Jacob of a concentration camp. Her experience under the Nazis had likely induced, as a result of identification with the aggressor, murderous thoughts against her own child; these thoughts left a great burden of guilt that she was perhaps never able to resolve. As a victim, Jacob's mother might assimilate Nazi behavior, which she had then passed to her child. Thus another reason that Jacob could not mourn his father's death was that the power of life and death over others that marks the mental world of the perennial mourner became condensed for him with the Nazi power over life and death.

Unsurprisingly, then, Jacob proved unable to express appropriate emotion overtly. When he wept, he literally went through only the motions of crying. What made his crying spells so eerie was that although he displayed appropriate facial expressions and sometimes even tears, he made no sounds. After abruptly ceasing to "cry," he would inhale deeply and then resume talking, as though nothing had happened, after several false starts. It was not until Jacob described the sensation of having an iron hand around his neck during a crying spell, however, that the full significance of his inability to express emotion overtly became clear. His first association was the memory of his final view of his father; confined to an iron lung, the father had, in effect, borne an iron collar around his neck. Later, however, Jacob was able to relate the details of another relevant experience that, he had been told, had occurred when the family was in hiding.

His parents had rented the house in Belgium with the idea that it would only be necessary to hide for 2 to 4 weeks; the hiding period lengthened to 2 years. Jacob's family lived on the first floor of the house, another Jewish family lived on the second, and the owners lived on the ground floor with their large dog. The owner made a practice of scaring the Jews by declaring, "The Gestapo are here," in order to extort more money or belongings to sell for himself. Only once did the Gestapo actually come to the door, but on another occasion it appeared that they had come again. As the dog barked loudly, the infant Jacob began to wail; the noise was felt to threaten the lives of those in hiding, so his father decided to strangle him. It was soon discovered, however, that the Gestapo were not in fact at the door, and the father immediately allowed the baby to breathe again. Family stories circulated later reflected the father's effort to rid himself of the terrible guilt that must have attached to this episode; over and over, he declared to Jacob that he would never have given his son alive to the Nazis. But Jacob's father was not alone; Niederland (1961) reports other cases of strangling children in order to prevent them from betraying a hideout to the Gestapo.

It can be safely assumed that Jacob's family, in a sense, never left their sad hiding place. The father, who had become physically helpless, died in the captivity of his iron lung. The mother, at the time Jacob was in treatment, still lived within the confines of an undesirable and even dangerous section of a city. Although she dreamed of "fresh air," particularly for her child, her unconscious suggested that they would never leave "the camp." Her son remained helpless, trying by indirection to gain help, love, and security, but unable to receive gratification or to develop trust. He, too, lived in a world still peopled by persecuting Nazis and victimized Jews.

Jacob's Negative Therapeutic Reaction

Convinced that his Jewish identity had doomed him to a hopeless path, Jacob defeated anyone, including his therapist, who tried to help him. During his treatment, he displayed an uncanny ability to enlist the feelings of others on his behalf, while simultaneously retaining a deep conviction that efforts to help him would be unavailing. He adhered absolutely to his helplessness, experiencing repeated episodes of anxiety and acute depression, displaying great pessimism, and clearly feeling entitled to complain capaciously whenever he felt like it. On occasion, when frustrated and angry, he felt as if he were a Nazi—which, in turn, made him feel guilty and scared. Although desperately in need of intimacy and closeness with others, he tended to show self-defeating patterns of excessive expectation, which turned into bitter and despairing withdrawal when what was done for him failed to measure up to his expectations. His choice of wife had exemplified this hopeful but easily disappointed dependence: Her strength as an "active Zionist" had led him to fantasize about being "saved" by her, but after they were married, he felt disappointed and foiled her attempts to offer him solace. Repeated arguments and a moody, stormy tone characterized the union. The early shared helplessness of young and old family members alike had become part of his identity and, paradoxically, rendered any potential helper helpless.

There seems to be a similarity between patients like Jacob and those known to psychoanalysts as *negative therapeutic reactors*. Stanley Olinick's (1964) review of this syndrome indicates that among other factors, defenses are directed against expected inner loss and helpless regression to primary identification with the depressed mother. He writes,

> Inevitably the mother's resentful helplessness and overcompensating, possessive demands, and the infant's or child's impotent aggressiveness will reinforce each other, with the result that the child grows up to be a welter of contradictions: demanding, but so fearful of disappointment as to be spuriously independent and rejecting; apprehensive of intrusion, yet fearful of isolation; wanting love, but able only to command or buy its counterfeit, dependence on and from the partner. (pp. 544–545)

These characteristics were all evident in Jacob, whose mother must have often felt helpless indeed in the hostile world that surrounded his infancy. Such patients defend themselves against being dependent or being abandoned. Their egos cannot find a comfortable position in relation to the object that will permit either closeness without fear of the loss of the sense of self, or separation without fear of the loss of the object. Therefore, in their relationships with others, these patients constantly oscillate between a wish for and a dread of symbiotic fusion, on the one hand, and a wish for and a dread of separation, on the other.

Through their apparent inability to alter their situation, they covertly communicate their wish to be rescued. They then ward off the anxiety created by this wish with defensive aggression—a need to sabotage the helper in order to enforce a sense of separateness and independence. His early interactions with his mother made Jacob a candidate for being a perennial mourner—that is, someone who would not accept separation or abandonment, but would instead attempt to control his feeling of extreme ambivalence toward the representation of the lost object.

Jacob left treatment after abandoning his studies and taking a position elsewhere. Dr. Volkan last saw Jacob several decades ago and has heard nothing from him since.

Living Statues and Memorial Candles

Dr. Volkan felt that Jacob had stopped his treatment because, both consciously and unconsciously, he wanted to remain a "living statue," a term coined by Volkan (1979) to describe the situation of a Cypriot boy named "Savaş" whom he met in 1974. The boy—whose name, in Turkish, means "War"—was born on the island of Cyprus on December 25, 1963. At this time, a "hot" conflict was raging, in which Greeks living on the island were trying to achieve dominance over the Turks living there, in an effort to unite the island with Greece. The period is known in Cypriot Turkish history as "Bloody Christmas."

During Bloody Christmas, a Turkish woman who had been captured by the Cypriot Greeks—as were many of the other Turks living in mixed villages near Nicosia, the capital city—gave birth to a son in the Nicosia General Hospital. The newborn child was left in a crib with other Cypriot Turkish infants who happened to be at this hospital—which, by then, was under total Cypriot Greek control. Horribly, the room where these infants were kept was also being used as a morgue for Cypriot Turks who had been killed in the fighting, but a British nurse, shocked by this situation, managed to separate the living infants from the dead adults. Two weeks later, the captured woman and her newborn son were allowed to leave the hospital and were brought, under the protection of the Red Cross, to the Turkish section of Nicosia, where the child's survival was hailed as a kind of miracle.

The infant's father, Özker Yaşın, was then a well-known poet. Upon his family's return to the Turkish section, he named his son "Savaş" and began writing a series of poems which were published later under the title *Letters to My Son Savas* (Yaşın, 1965). A poetic history of the Cyprus conflict for the two years beginning with Savaş's birth, as seen from the point of view of a Cypriot Turk, *Letters* begins with a description of the events taking place at the time that the boy named "War" "was opening his eyes on the world" (p. 18). It conveys a sense that the poet's child was immortal—or at least, a very special being:

With a bullet from a lowly person
You could have died, Savaş,
Before you were born:
You could die in your mother's belly
Without getting to know
The miracle called life
Thanks to which you were saved. (p. 18)

When Dr. Volkan conducted clinical interviews with Savaş, then age 11, it was clear that his parents' and others' perception of him—and his own unconscious fantasy of himself—as the symbol of Bloody Christmas had become part of the boy's self-representation, causing him to develop an obsessional personality. As a symbol, Savaş felt it was necessary for him to be perfect in order to meet the expectations of his father and of those his father had reached with his stirring poetry. One of his most telling presenting symptoms was an odd sensation of dryness in the skin of his face; he thought if he scratched it, parts of his countenance would chip off as though from the face of a stone statue. In his unconscious fantasy, the boy named "War" was a national monument, a "living statue."

Dina Wardi (1992), who conducted individual and group therapy with many children of Holocaust survivors in Israel, noted that many of them expressed the feeling that they occupied a special place on earth. During her work, when they were between the ages of 25 and 35, they were, like Savaş, living flags symbolizing their large group's identity. Wardi dubbed such individuals *memorial candles*. Because the offspring of survivors had a special task to perform—a task that rightfully belonged to their parents and their large group—they exhibited difficulties in their separation-individuation processes. And, like Jacob, they would most likely have difficulty in mourning when facing object losses. Wardi writes, "It is thus not surprising that these sons and daughters, who sense their special place in their family and their value for their parents, also find it very difficult in the end to separate [intrapsychically] from their parents and liberate themselves from their difficult tasks" (p. 34). Wardi noted, too, that many of these "memorial candles" were replacement children, perceived by their parents as representing relatives who had perished during the Holocaust. Some sons and daughters "were given multiple names as [if] they were supposed to carry the whole family around on their shoulders" (p. 28). Within an individual family, she noted, other siblings could be freed from the heavy burden of the Holocaust legacy if one child were "chosen" to be the "memorial candle."

In his unconscious fantasy, Jacob, too, was a living statue or memorial candle for whom there could be "no exit" into further psychological development. When Dr. Volkan presented Jacob's case to colleagues at a professional meeting while Jacob was still in treatment, a Jewish psychoanalyst in the audience became upset. He, too, declared Jacob a living memorial and told Dr. Volkan not to tamper with such a special being. As a living statue, Jacob belonged to his large group; as a living memorial, he contained the legacy of the Third Reich, including the identities of both the Jews and the Nazis. The process of mourning would modify his self-concept, including the images of his persecuted parents for which he had become a reservoir. But Jacob would not mourn, and thus remained a living statue.

6

Leo

A JEWISH MAN LIVING IN TWO WORLDS

IN THE CLINICAL LITERATURE on second-generation Holocaust survivors, cases like Jacob's are typical, insofar as most patients' parents were either helpless victims or death camp survivors (Jacob's is somewhat unique, in that he was himself an infant survivor, as well as the child of survivors). The father of the patient whose case we report in this chapter, however, was neither of these. Entreated by relatives in Germany to help them escape the Nazis, he bravely obtained a visa to travel to Germany, where he passed himself off as a gentile. Of course, if his deception had been discovered, he might have been killed; survival under these circumstances obviously depended upon his hypervigilance. Under such extreme conditions, we surmise, he internalized and assimilated not only the perilous nature of the external world, but also the role of the aggressor. Moreover, after he left this world of genuine danger, he seems to have maintained the defensive adaptations he had developed and later passed them to his son, Leo, who was a physician in his early 40s when he entered treatment with Dr. Greer. Images of his father's experiences under the Third Reich permeated every aspect of Leo's internalized object relations and psychosexual development. Unwittingly, Leo had become a protagonist in his father's drama; in Leo's unconscious fantasies, his past had become so inextricably intertwined with his father's traumatic past that he constantly lived in two worlds—his own and that of his father.

Leo's Parents' History: Courage and Cowardice

Leo's paternal grandparents were liberal Central European immigrants to the United States who were able to raise their son, Leo's father, under relatively affluent circumstances. Leo has only vague memories of his grandfather as a meek person who, as a cantor, was deeply involved in the Jewish community in the major eastern U.S. city where they lived. An intelligent young man, Leo's father graduated with honors from a prestigious university and went on to an equally well-respected law school, where he soon distinguished himself as a legal scholar. After law school, he traveled to Britain, where he studied economics at a world-renowned institution.

During the father's time in Britain Adolf Hitler rose to power, and it was bruited in the city where Leo's father lived that Jews were being persecuted in Germany. Since German Jews had been loyal to the Kaiser during World War I, this report was difficult for many Jews outside of Germany—including Leo's father—to credit, but relatives living in Germany soon confirmed the rumors. Courageously, he responded to their desperate pleas by surreptitiously entering Germany to arrange their escape. Because his surname could also be German and because he spoke German fluently, he was able to masquerade as a gentile. As Leo related this part of his father's story, he interjected that the non-Jews with whom his father was associated "would have been thrilled" to kill him. Leo did not know whether or not any relatives were saved, but believes that most of his father's family in Germany and other Nazi-occupied countries were killed.

Because our information comes from Leo himself, we have few details about the father's activities in Germany as he moved "freely" about the country as a non-Jew. But it is obvious that at his own peril, Leo's father was involved in activities extremely unusual for a Jew. For instance, while attending a rally in Nuremberg, he saw Hitler deliver a speech to a throng of partisans. Although we do not know why Leo's father would choose to attend a major Nazi event, he must have pretended that he was a Nazi himself in order to keep his Jewish identity unsuspected. Based on skeletal anecdotes such as this one, we believe that Leo's father was probably required on a number of occasions to "become" not merely a non-Jew but actually a "Nazi."

Several years after returning to the United States, he was admitted to a psychiatric hospital and diagnosed as "paranoid schizophrenic." No treatment records of Leo's father's hospitalization have been available to Leo or to us. Given the fact that even in Israel, Holocaust survivors were admitted to mental hospitals without any reference to the fact that they had endured an inconceivable horror, however, we would not be surprised if, upon inspection, his treatment records revealed no mention of the fact that paranoia had been a necessary condition of survival in this man's past reality. Surely, he had internalized, under a most stressful situation, a paranoid environment.

Leo's father and mother were married after his father's daring ventures into Nazi Germany, and Leo was born five years after the end of World War II. Other than these scant facts, Leo knew nothing about this epochal period of his father's life; it had been shrouded in a veil of silence. Nevertheless, as a child, Leo experienced his father as an already "profoundly changed" man. Though he knew of his father's gallantry in Germany, young Leo perceived his father as a "coward," someone who seemed constantly terrified. When most people might feel anger or some other appropriate affect, his father would feel panic. Formerly a sociable, amiable, and vivacious person with many friends, Leo's father had become a highly suspicious "recluse" with unconventional political beliefs.

Leo's parents' political affiliation with the Communist Party in an era of virulent anticommunism in the United States made it very difficult for his father to get a job. The family was dogged by the FBI throughout the McCarthy era; Bureau agents even purportedly tapped the family's telephone. By this time, however, his father had been deemed a "paranoid schizophrenic" by the medical establishment. Leo's mother told him that his father suffered from visual hallucinations and delusional beliefs. Among these, Leo's father felt that she was poisoning him and that he was being persecuted by Fascists. Only during Leo's analysis did he realize that his perceptions of his father were tainted by his mother's continual denigration of her ex-husband as a feckless coward.

After the demise of McCarthyism in the mid-1950s, Leo's parents' marriage disintegrated, and they divorced when Leo was 7 years old. Leo's father obtained a faculty position at a college in the Northeast, far away from his ex-wife and sons, but telephoned his children weekly. Leo and his older brother spent part of their summer holidays with their father. Leo continued to visit his father annually until he was 15 years old, but never learned much about his father's life in Nazi Germany. Leo's father moved around the United States "like a Gypsy," as Leo puts it, before finally settling on the West Coast as a university professor. When Leo was 20, his father remarried; Leo calls his stepmother a "good and sensitive" woman.

Leo's father periodically invited his sons to join him and his new wife for vacations. On one trip during Leo's early 20s, he and his brother crewed for the older man on a sailing trip that went awry. When they encountered a dangerous situation, Leo's father became so frightened that he abandoned the sailboat in a dinghy by himself, leaving his sons at the helm. Leo and his brother managed to sail the boat to safety, later picking up their father at the shore. Both vowed never to crew for their father again, and they never did. After this incident, Leo shunned his father as a "coward," for all practical purposes avoiding any contact with the man. After Leo himself was married for the first time in his mid-20s, his father, now retired, moved to the city where Leo had settled. Still, Leo kept his distance from his father, who died when Leo was 40 years old.

We wish we had more information about Leo's father. Although Dr. Greer suspected from the first that the father's experiences in Nazi Germany had affected Leo's internal world, it was only as their work together progressed that the profound influence of his father's Third Reich–related self- and object-images began to become evident in Leo's unconscious fantasies. In these fantasies, Leo and the persons to whom he related intimately were alternately aggressive and omnipotent Nazis and "cowardly" Jewish victims doomed to hypervigilance. If they expressed their rage fully, they could kill; if they showed their vulnerability, they could be killed.

It would be most interesting as well to understand more fully the psychodynamics of Leo's parents' marriage, including why, as Leo perceived it, his father passively accepted his first wife's verbal and physical abuse. Did he feel guilty for not being able to save his Jewish relatives in Germany and other Nazi-occupied territories? Was he perhaps identifying with those endangered relatives in order to appease his guilt? Or did he feel so crushed under Nazi might that in the long run, he surrendered his former courage, resigning himself to a hazardous home environment so that he could hold onto his "paranoid" identity? Did he marry Leo's mother to help him create a dangerous—Nazi—world?

Of course, we will never have direct answers to such questions, just as we will never know directly why Leo's mother, who came from a wealthy American Jewish family involved in the silk industry, chose his father. Did she feel guilty for the lavish lifestyle she had enjoyed while her people—and perhaps her relatives—suffered under the Nazis in Europe? We know that later in life she joined her husband in the Communist Party, and she voluntarily gave up luxury on many occasions. As a child and a young woman, she had worn silk garments; as an adult, she refused to wear silk and went about in what Leo described as "sackcloth and ashes." Was she rebelling against her parents, whom she reviled as unscrupulous capitalists, or was she also trying to identify with suffering Jews? We simply cannot know the answers.

Leo's Life Story: Maternal Abuse and a Failed Psychoanalysis

What we do know is that Leo's mother exhibited extreme aggression toward her husband and sons, creating a chillingly traumatic developmental period for Leo. Leo recalled paroxysms of rage in which she would strike out at him and migraine headaches during which she would retreat to bed, insisting that she not be disturbed. She beat Leo with wire coat hangers, wooden clothes brushes, and a leather strap. If there were no implements available with which to beat him, she grabbed him by the hair and pulled it as hard as she could. Leo recalls that on several occasions she told him, "I could cut your throat with pleasure." Leo reports that he was 30 years old before he realized, after seeing how humanely his friends treated their own children, that he had been a victim of child abuse.

His father, who was not physically abusive, was still an object of fear and anxiety throughout Leo's childhood and adolescence. During summer vacations, the father showed more attention to his older son and played little with Leo. Leo's brother was always permitted to ride in the front seat of the car, and when the younger son attempted to communicate with his father from the back seat, Leo remembers, his father ignored him as if he did not exist. Leo's paternal grandmother also came to visit her son during the summers but paid little attention to Leo, so preoccupied was she with Leo's father. Leo does recall, however, some happy and secure childhood moments with his father, including sucking his thumb while sitting on his father's lap. And when Leo was 12 years old, his father came to the city where Leo and his brother lived with their mother, in order to attend Leo's Bar Mitzvah. Though he remembers his father hugging him tightly, Leo consciously did not wish his father to be at the ceremony and continued to see the man as "crazy." As will be described later, Leo's relationship with his mother was so intense and so full of separation-individuation difficulties (Mahler, 1968) that in his oedipal fantasies, his father was perceived either as a scary ("crazy") person or as a devalued one. In the absence of maternal abuse, the events in the car, for instance, would not have been so laden with meaning for Leo; he would have been able to appreciate the loving things his father tried to do for him, rather than focusing on the father's anxiety-producing actions. Instead, Leo had no opportunity to move normally up the development ladder, even if his father had actually behaved "normally."

Unsurprisingly, Leo was an extremely anxious child, often sucking his thumb and suffering psychosomatic symptoms. After his father left behind their chaotic family life, Leo learned to fend for himself during his mother's sudden temporary desertions. As she impetuously left her sons by themselves, sometimes for a week or more, Leo began to prepare his own meals. He was unable to read until the third grade and was diagnosed with dyslexia. As a boy, he was taunted and abused by his peers: He was a victim. As a teenager, however, he attempted to identify with the "brave" father image. In high school, he bicycled across the country with several friends, a feat on which he prided himself for his "courage." When he was in college, Leo flew to Europe by himself, hitchhiked around the continent, and learned enough German and French to communicate easily with the local population. We see this trip as another symbolic attempt to identify with the father who had ventured into Nazi Germany.

Notwithstanding their abusive family background and despite their modest financial circumstances, both Leo and his brother, who is 3 years older, were able to pursue higher education. Leo's brother, however, fell apart in college. Though he managed to become an architect, he sabotaged his own success, becoming deeply involved in drugs and frequenting prostitutes. Leo, as an adult, scorned his brother as a sociopath. When Leo himself went to college and then to medical school, he took pride in his own self-sufficiency and competence. Shocked by how many of his fellow students were unable to prepare meals or do their own laundry, Leo overtly felt superior to others, already exhibiting a narcissistic personality organization. Covertly, however, he remained a dependent victim.

After completing his internship, Leo married, but soon came to perceive his new wife as dangerous and felt he could not trust her. In analysis, he stated that she had undergone a "metamorphosis" after they were married by becoming an alcoholic; the untrustworthy and dangerous environment that Leo expected had become a reality. Once, while Leo was on call at the hospital, his wife was brought to the emergency room in handcuffs by the police for public intoxication. On another occasion, in an intoxicated state, she brandished a pistol at Leo. Later, on hearing how Leo related to "his women," Dr. Greer came to believe that, in fact, Leo had played a substantial role in recreating the unsafe, "paranoia"-inducing environment that his father had suffered during marriage to Leo's mother. Leo threatened to leave his wife if she did not get help and did so when she refused, just six months after they were married.

After they separated, Leo had numerous "meaningless affairs." He prided himself in his ability to discern these women's "defects and flaws." He wanted to "select" a woman who measured up to his exalted standards, but all he could find were, in his words, "defective women." On the occasions that Leo managed some self-reflection during this period, he wondered if the problem lay within himself. He briefly saw two psychiatrists, both of whom he found to be "unsatisfactory." Eventually, he met a "gentle" Jewish woman with whom he lived for 5 years; finally, however, he found sex with her "dreadful" and ended the relationship. Later, Leo became involved with another woman, a gentile, and they married. Predictably, she, too, was soon perceived as a threat; her outbursts scared him.

In order to answer his questions about women and marriage, Leo sought help from a psychoanalyst several years prior to this second marriage. After 4 years of analysis on a 4 times per week basis, he developed extremely negative feelings for his analyst; the analyst, in turn, became so exasperated with his patient's relentless aggression toward him that he abruptly discontinued their work together, granting Leo only two sessions to terminate. Leo was humiliated, enraged, and flooded with daydreams of revenge for his dismissal from analysis. In spite of the many irregularities of his first analysis, Leo would eventually come to feel that he had benefited from the experience, which, to some extent, may be true. Leo and his analyst had, in a sense, recreated the patient's early environment, a space of verbal abuse and continual boundary violation; in reality, however, what they had created was indeed safer than the original anarchy of Leo's family life. In a sense, then, this exercise allowed the patient to discharge rage and other feelings related to his early childhood environment. Nevertheless, such a "treatment" could not lead to meaningful structural changes in the patient's psychic life. Shortly after this fiasco, Leo began analysis with Dr. Greer in order to understand what had happened with his previous analysis and to continue trying to understand himself.

Overcoming the "Built-In Transference"

It was clear to Dr. Greer from the beginning of his work with Leo that the patient had come to him with a "built-in transference": an unresolved transference (and in many cases, a transference neurosis) developed with a previous therapist and brought to a new analyst when the prior analytical work is abruptly terminated. Because these premature transference phenomena (Werman, 1984) appear so early in analysis, before the new analyst fully understands the patient's psychodynamics, they are easily misinterpreted. Until the feelings, attitudes, and fantasies that have been suddenly and massively transferred to the new analyst are correctly understood and worked through, however, the patient can initiate no genuine therapeutic alliance with the new analyst.

Aware of the potential for a built-in transference in this case, Dr. Greer began by nonjudgmentally listening to Leo speak about his previous analysis, which appeared to have been chaotic, especially in its later phases. For instance, the previous analyst frequently used Leo's analytic sessions to discuss the symptoms of patients whom Leo had referred to the analyst. Leo, in turn, began to bring an alarm clock to his sessions to ensure that the analyst would neither cheat him nor overrun the time allotted. The analyst was apparently oblivious to this derivative of Leo's internal "alarm"; his deviation from the standard analytic framework magnified Leo's transference expectation of a dangerous intimate environment, which would have appeared under any analytical circumstances. Continual boundary violations compromised the background of safety (Sandler, 1960) crucial to successful analysis, and soon the analyst and the patient were screaming at each other, with the analyst allegedly calling his patient "sadistic, manipulative, or borderline." Of course, we do not know Leo's previous analyst personally, nor do we know his usual manner of treatment. What Leo told Dr. Greer about his previous analyst is likely to have contained transferential distortions and expressions of Leo's own personality organization. At the least, however, it seems clear that both parties invaded the therapeutic space repeatedly. Under these circumstances, Leo's analysis came to a premature end.

When Dr. Greer did not validate Leo's harangue, Leo called Dr. Greer "incompetent," as if he were an extension of the previous analyst, and launched a relentless attack on his new therapist. Indeed, Leo's attacks were so insistent that at times Dr. Greer thought that perhaps Leo's previous analyst had correctly assessed Leo as unanalyzable. Dr. Greer managed to maintain his therapeutic position in the face of Leo's aggression, however, and did not allow himself to be drawn into an aggressive counter-action. Before long, the attacks tempered; leaving Dr. Greer's office, Leo would smile and say, "Just fucking with you," as if to reassure the analyst that he was merely being tested. Eventually, Dr. Greer pondered with Leo the idea that perhaps he was anxious that his new analyst, like the previous one, would "throw him out" for being so aggressive. When Dr. Greer encouraged him to verbalize such fears rather than enact them, Leo recalled that his maternal grandmother had nicknamed him the German epithet *Fres*, "wild animal."

Noting Leo's extreme wariness and his use of a German word to designate his aggressive self, Dr. Greer pointed out that hypervigilance would have been a highly adaptive response for Leo's father as he moved among the Nazis. Perhaps, Dr. Greer suggested, Leo identified with the image of his father in imminent danger of detection. Furthermore, the abuse that Leo had suffered as a child might incline him to identify with the image of a hypervigilant father. Leo was surprised and intrigued by the analyst's remarks; none of his previous three therapists had linked his behavior patterns with the father's experiences in Nazi Germany. Indeed, as would become clear, Leo's prior analyst seemed to have actively avoided the topic, even though Leo had told the analyst his father's story and even though the previous analyst himself is Jewish.

Leo now began to differentiate Dr. Greer from his previous analyst, while pouring out more childhood recollections. He recalled with emotion that when he was only 4 years old, his mother repeatedly left him alone in the car while she shopped in the city. When she would return to discover him in tears of terror, the mother would scold rather than comfort her son. Often Leo would "balance" such recollections of childhood helplessness by demonstrations of his self-sufficiency in adapting to early traumas: how, for example, at the age of 9 years, he fearlessly traveled by himself from the suburbs where he lived with his mother and brother into the city.

Since Leo had been in analysis for 4 years before becoming Dr. Greer's patient, he readily saw certain connections between his present behavior patterns and his childhood experiences. He had a strong sense that his troubles with women had a great deal to do with his childhood experiences of his mother. He was also concerned that he had inherited what he called his father's "biological disease": his paranoid schizophrenia, which Leo understood as a genetic medical condition without regard or empathy for the father's extremely anxiety-provoking experiences under the Third Reich. Leo reported that he knew himself to be "paranoid" because he had "a radar that reaches the horizon. I see danger long before it becomes evident to others." Once Dr. Greer suggested to Leo that his father might also have passed on to him images of the Nazis and their victims, Leo soon began to illustrate clearly the intertwining of Nazi images with his own developmental object relations and psychosexual conflicts.

Early Illustrations of "This Nazi/Jewish Stuff"

When Leo entered analysis with Dr. Greer, he had been married to his second wife for one year. They had discovered that she was infertile, and she was taking a fertility drug that could result in multiple births, a prospect that consciously concerned Leo because of the danger of renal failure for his wife. Dr. Greer sensed, however, that the matter of becoming a parent carried other meanings for Leo as well. He wished to have children, but this wish seemed to clash with an unconscious fear that the children, as extensions of him, would face a dangerous world. Thus, covertly, he was determined not to have children. Because the analyst did not know at this point whether the question of having children was also overshadowed by fantasies concerning the fate of Jewish children in Nazi Germany, he did not yet mention this possibility to his patient.

As their work together progressed, however, other aspects of Leo's inner world began to reveal themselves as Nazi-identified. As the patient described his conflicted sexual and emotional relationship with his wife, Dr. Greer came to understand that Leo used his sexual organ as if it were a "fecal penis," full of sadism. Recalling Leo's previous selection of women with "defects," Dr. Greer noted that during sex with them, Leo had felt no affection; he wanted only to discharge his rage and to "shoot scum up" in their genitals, as he put it. Leo's perceptions of these women were much like Nazis' assessments of the women they used (if illegally) for sex and for "scientific" experiments; both considered the women they exploited less than human.

Toward the end of the third month of his work with Dr. Greer, the relationship between Leo and his wife became extremely violent. As the rancor escalated between them, Leo experienced conscious wishes to kill his wife. These murderous thoughts were accompanied by disclaimers that he would ever act upon such impulses, an attempt to reassure both himself and his analyst that he was not really homicidal. Leo's wife, in turn, became more volatile and aggressive toward him. At such times, in his words, she would become a "storm trooper." Leo dreaded falling, as he said, "victim to a predator." He dreamed of himself as helpless, clad in a black hood and attacked by an executioner, a dream that echoed an adolescent experience in which Leo was attacked from behind by another boy. In reality, as he was being choked, Leo panicked, but nevertheless managed to break the boy's hold and escape. Leo reported, too, that the image of himself in the dream reminded him of Jews being gassed in Nazi camps. Dr. Greer reminded Leo that the analyst himself was sitting *behind* the patient and that analytic work itself might cause anxiety as well. Dr. Greer's suggestion that Leo might be using Nazi and Holocaust images to express his anxiety about the analyst's power made Leo feel, as he said, "understood for the first time."

Leo then revealed an intense interest in European history—German history, in particular. His extemporaneous discourses on European history over the course of his analysis were impressive for their erudition and detail. Leo's vast knowledge of the social, political, and military history of many European peoples—especially the Germans—from classical times to the present was remarkable for a nonhistorian. Soon, Leo's hours were filled with his account of the creation of the modern German state and German Jews' significant role in this process. During these lectures, Leo periodically broke out into an SS song, which reminded Dr. Greer of Leo's father attending the Nuremberg rally in order to hide his identity and intentions. Leo's SS songs on the couch on one level thus illustrated his (or his father's) "identification" with the Nazis. Leo also seemed, however, to be mocking the Nazis with his singing: a kind of *opéra bouffe*.

Dr. Greer is himself a history buff, but he noted immediately that his knowledge of European history, especially of the Nazi period, paled in comparison to Leo's. By exhibiting his superior knowledge, Leo was, in a sense, trying to devalue his analyst. Dr. Greer resisted the counter-reaction of being forced to "lose" an intellectual competition with a patient; his feeling of disquietude had a deeper meaning. When Leo began to interject foreign phrases—phrases with which Dr. Greer was not likely to be, and indeed was not, familiar—into the "lectures," Dr. Greer came to see that he was, to Leo, like a fledgling student; he was Leo's father in a foreign (German) land, listening to SS songs and not knowing the nuances of the (Nazi) language. Leo had externalized the deposited image of his father in Dr. Greer. The analyst's countertransference response and his understanding of its deeper meaning (Boyer, 1983, 1999), with which it was not necessary to burden his patient, provided additional evidence that the patient had indeed been a reservoir for the father's anxious self-images.

Another anecdote revealed the ambivalence in Leo's "educative" gestures. While interning in an American city with a large German population—which, he now disclosed for the first time, he had chosen in conscious imitation of his father—he had shared an interest in German history with another authority figure. Because Leo's surname did not betray his ethnic background as a Jew, his supervisors assumed he was a gentile, and he never told them otherwise. One of his supervisors was so impressed with Leo's extensive knowledge of German history that the man offered him a staff position when he completed his internship. Believing that Leo was a gentile—as the Nazis presumably had believed that Leo's father was a gentile—this man then loaned him a volume about the notorious SS division that executed American captives at the Battle of the Bulge. In truth, as Leo learned, this man had been born and raised in Nazi Germany and might well have been a Nazi himself. Unsurprisingly, Leo reported having felt "nervous" during his whole tenure under this man's supervision. Perhaps now Leo was once more identifying directly with his father, anxiously proving his knowledge to the potentially dangerous, possibly Nazi authority figure, his analyst.

Around this time, Leo visited the Holocaust Museum in Washington, D.C., for the first time. Although he did not speak of his reactions to the museum during his sessions, he told Dr. Greer in the weeks that followed that "this Nazi/Jewish stuff" was beginning to make sense to him. Referring to his wife as a "bad mother" *and* as a Nazi, he vowed to turn his "radar on" and attempted to make "preemptive strikes" against her. On guard at all times against "being trashed or got rid of," he sought a divorce, consulting three "killer attorneys" chosen for their reputedly aggressive court behavior. In daydreams around this time, Leo envisioned Hitler at the Eagle's Nest, the Führer's retreat in the Bavarian Alps, signifying an identification with the Nazi leader quite literally at the "height" of his power. Soon after the daydream, Leo took his loaded handgun, which he had kept at home in a secure place, and left it on the marital bed, where his wife found it. Though this gesture clearly functioned as a threat, reflecting Leo's identification with Nazi murderers, leaving the gun on the bed also left Leo open to the fear that his wife would shoot him, signaling an identification with Jewish victims.

As he "Nazi-fied" himself openly, he began to fear that Dr. Greer, like his previous analyst, would turn against him, a concern that Dr. Greer was able to use to defuse the potentially violent situation that Leo had created. Reiterating that Leo was reenacting the conflicts of his childhood with his parents through Third Reich images, Dr. Greer told Leo that there was no room for a loaded gun in the therapeutic process, that it was imperative that he put his wishes and anxieties into words in an atmosphere where aggressive impulses could safely be discussed and lead to insights. Leo responded not merely by unloading the handgun and putting it away, but by becoming preoccupied with Winston Churchill's volumes of World War II history. By handling the handgun issue directly, Dr. Greer had, in a sense, become Churchill—the man who would rescue Leo (in his victim-identification) from the "Nazi" wife. Paradoxically, because he felt more secure with Dr. Greer, Leo now transferred his full sadism toward his therapist, which gave some relief to his wife. Because Dr. Greer did not respond to his behavior as had the previous analyst—who, when subjected to Leo's sadism, would tell the patient that he had a "bad prognosis"—Leo was further differentiating Dr. Greer as a "new object."

* * *

As his wife announced that she was going to leave him, Leo suddenly remembered an incident that had occurred on board a cruise ship when he was 10 years old. It was another occasion on which Leo's father had invited his sons to join him for a holiday. Leo was playing ping-pong when a female passenger in her early 20s asked if she could play. He refused, and when she tried to grab the paddle from his hand, he punched her in the eye. Much to Leo's surprise, her husband failed to intercede, but the woman herself managed to wrestle Leo down and turned him over to a member of the ship's staff for discipline. Focusing on the husband's inaction, Leo found a parallel between the woman's husband and his own father, who had never taught him the rules of appropriate social conduct. Dr. Greer suggested to Leo that perhaps his father had indirectly communicated to him that if he were to survive in a Nazi world, he must be a Nazi himself; if one were a Nazi, one would be immune from the rules that ordinarily govern social behavior. During this time of his analysis, Leo had begun to interject "correct me if I'm wrong" whenever he expressed an opinion. Calling this speech pattern to Leo's attention, Dr. Greer suggested that his request to be corrected might represent his lack, in childhood, of a father to teach him right from wrong. After internalizing Nazi Germany, perhaps his father could not supply moral education or tame Leo's aggression, especially toward women whom he perceived as abusing or rejecting him. Leo then recalled having behaved violently to animals during his childhood, once squeezing a guinea pig so hard that he injured it. His childhood rage at times made him feel shame, but most often scared him.

As Leo and his wife separated, Dr. Greer observed that Leo did not know how to deal with a loss and the anger that accompanied it; the patient frequently expressed himself in Nazi images and other aggressive acts so as not to experience his covert dependent side. Leo reported that his answering machine now had a Wagner opera on it, emphasizing Wagner's place in Nazi iconography, and envisaged himself coming to analysis in jackboots and a field gray Nazi uniform. Before his wife took her clothes from the house they had shared, he ejaculated into his wife's underwear when she was absent and then poured bleach on them.

Several weeks after she moved out, Leo shamefully reported that he had wet the bed. He felt utterly humiliated, saying that he would be careful to empty his bladder from now on before going to bed. As he pondered this symptom in analysis, he remembered an incident that had occurred when he was a small boy. While in the bathtub, he thought that he had to flatulate, but defecated instead. His mother had berated him mercilessly. The next session began with Leo asking Dr. Greer, "Do you care if I smell?" as if he had brought the memory of defecating in the bathtub back with him to the session; Leo was now going to reveal the most aggressive aspects of himself. In a child's mind, there are "good" and "bad" smells, the "bad" primarily belonging to the child's anal sadism. Associating to the memory of humiliation, Leo said that he wanted to believe that Dr. Greer had developed an attachment to him. "I want you to care about me as I wished my parents had cared for me," he said wistfully. When Leo revealed that he had discontinued a soporific he had been taking since his wife left, Dr. Greer commented that perhaps he was prepared to show both of them his "shitty" side.

In response, Leo reported that the previous evening he had gone out with a woman whom he had "banged." After sex, he had noticed that the condom had a tear in it and that, much to his dismay, he did indeed have active herpes, though he had checked himself prior to their encounter. He rebuked himself for being so thoughtless as to have possibly infected the woman. Dr. Greer suggested to Leo that beneath his ostensible concern for this woman was an unadulterated aggression that was displaced from the image of his mother, and that Leo perceived himself as a Nazi who used Jewish women without regard for their health or needs. Leo admitted that he could be an aggressive, dirty, fecal person; the idea that he "blasted" women with a "dirty" penis was difficult for him to own, however. He then recalled a dream in which he saw a face with a large detachable nose that looked "like the devil incarnate" and suggested that the image condensed the images of Jew and Nazi with which he alternately identified. The nose also stood for his "dirty" penis—which, since it was detachable, he could own or disown according to the circumstances. The castration anxiety that would be primary for many patients in such a dream was left in the background, as he struggled with anxieties surrounding his identity.

He then disclosed something that he had withheld for several months:

When his wife had come to pick up her clothes, they had quarreled and he had pushed her down; she had brought charges against Leo for assault and battery, which, he was elated to report, had just been dismissed. When he lost control of himself, he said, "I *became* a Nazi." Using Nazi images to defend himself against knowing his dependency needs led Leo to recall a "Nazi phase" in his adolescence during which he caricatured the Nazi goosestep and wore "biker clothes." When police officers saw him in public, they shadowed him closely, as if he were a potential one-man crime spree. He also began to use drugs and would stay high for days at a time while his mother was gone, though he eventually gave up the drug use and never became an addict. Because Leo could not travel normally through adolescence, a phase during which an internal review of the youngster's investment in childhood self- and object-images takes place and some images are modified or given up, he had been unable to let go of or change the childhood images of his mother, his father, and himself. His "Nazi phase," which ended in his late teens, had been a defensive response to this inability. By the beginning of Leo's second year of treatment with Dr. Greer, Leo could more openly concede that the idea that his father's traumatized images had influenced his own mental development was an invaluable conceptual tool that explained much about him that he had not understood. Now, he reported, he could see the "shadows of Nazis all over my life."

Not long thereafter, Leo was notified by an aunt that his mother, who lived in another city, had developed an inoperable brain tumor. He briefly considered offering his medical expertise to assist in her care; he thought that perhaps they might even reconcile before she died. But he reasoned that even if she did change, he could never get what he wanted from her because he was no longer a child. "What I want," he said, "is childish": for her to see him as a lovable son, for her to love him. Fearing that what he called his "dark side" might erupt, he resolutely decided not to assist in her care or even to visit her. If they met, there might be murder; either he would act out his rage and kill her, or he would submit to her, this "Nazi" woman. With gallows humor, Leo quipped that if he did go to see his mother, it would probably be after she died, and then only to see if they draped a swastika over her coffin. He could not simply visit with her before she died.

Before Leo learned of his mother's terminal illness, he continued to drift from woman to woman as he had done since his second divorce. He acknowledged that he missed his ex-wife, but not what he called her "craziness"; he began to date younger women without "too much baggage." Now Leo's wish to escape preoccupation with his ill mother made him enamored with Diana, a woman in her 20s. Though he was concerned about the propriety of their substantial age difference, he initially felt more comfortable with Diana than with any woman with whom he had been involved in the past. Describing her as attractive and pleasant, he was particularly captivated by Diana's kindness and lack of aggression; indeed, he idealized her. Soon, however, Leo could not manage to keep the image of Diana from becoming contaminated with the image of his mother. He began to fear that she would turn into a "monster." When he became ill with influenza, he complained about Diana's purported lack of concern and dreamed of being chased by a prehistoric creature that represented the archaic image of his bad mother. Comparing himself to Henry Higgins who, in the G. B. Shaw play *Pygmalion*, molds a street flower vendor into the woman of his dreams, Leo even considered "training" Diana for "good" qualities.

Leo's quest to create a "good" mother before his biological mother died was also observable in the transference. An epicure who loved fine food and wines, Leo began to recite recipes for various gourmet dishes he had prepared. Eventually, Leo asked Dr. Greer whether he wrote any of these recipes down and, if so, whether he had tried any of them yet. In his regressed state, Leo had become a nurturing parent, while Dr. Greer represented a child needing to be cared for and fed. In a dream around this time, Leo found himself eating a tuna fish sandwich that had ceramic plates for bread; in association, the dream recalled for him how bad a cook his mother had been when he was a child. For instance, she had frequently left shards of eggshell in his eggs despite his complaints. He had thought at times that she intentionally sabotaged his food to torment him, and, consequently, he had begun to prepare his own meals at a very young age. It now occurred to him that this experience might bear on the question of why he preferred to do as much of the "interpretive" work for himself as possible in his treatment. Perhaps only then, in his mind, could he be sure that the analytical work would be done properly. But neither Leo's attempt to mother Dr. Greer nor his effort to create a nonaggressive woman in Diana could be sustained for very long.

Hours during which Leo could find links between his childhood experiences and present relationships with others, including Dr. Greer, often alternated with sessions in which Leo evoked images of the Third Reich to recall and reenact his childhood. As, in anticipation of his mother's death, he contemplated the depth of her murderous rage toward him and his murderous rage toward her, Leo's mind was populated with Nazis. In a dream from this time, he was sitting on a bench with a group of people he identified as Christians, staring at shops with broken windows. Realizing that his companions were neo-Nazis, he looked down and noticed that he himself was wearing jackboots. For Leo, the dream recalled *Kristallnacht*, the 1938 "Night of Broken Glass," a two-night rampage in which Nazis attacked Jews and ransacked synagogues, Jewish cemeteries, schools, and Jewish-owned shops in Germany, Austria, and the Sudetenland.

Nazis and Vampires

As Leo's mother's illness progressed, derivatives of a particular unconscious fantasy surfaced; as became clear, this fantasy condensed the Nazi self-image that appeared in the *Kristallnacht* dream with Leo's oral sadism against his mother and, in turn, her oral sadism against him. First, Leo recalled a New Year's Eve in his late teens when he had dressed up as a vampire. With other revelers at a party, he had gone to a wax museum, where he pretended to be a mannequin; when visitors approached, he lunged at them. He then jumped up suddenly from the couch to illustrate this stunt for Dr. Greer; naturally, like some of the museum visitors, Dr. Greer was startled. After Leo returned to the couch and Dr. Greer regained his composure, Leo remembered that as a child, he had once bitten his mother and that his mother had bitten him back. Thus, in fantasy, either Leo or his mother could be a vampire. Continuing to explore the New Year's Eve event, Leo remembered that a few years before the incident in the wax museum, he had gone through a phase in which he was overtly phobic about vampires and werewolves. As he explained to Dr. Greer that he had known how to keep vampires away, he realized that Jewish–Christian issues were condensed with his phobia: one could save oneself from a vampire by holding onto a cross—that is, by being a Christian. Leo's associations then turned to the swastika, the Nazi cross: he had to be a Christian/Nazi in order to protect himself from his projected oral sadism, represented by the vampire, which paradoxically was associated with Nazism itself. In his unconscious fantasy, then, Leo had to identify with the Nazis in order to avoid falling victim to them—just as his father had been forced to do in reality. We conclude that the deposited image of his Nazi-era father had initiated Leo's history-related unconscious fantasy.

Toward the end of Leo's second year of treatment with Dr. Greer, the news arrived that his mother had died. At his first session following her death, he sang, in his inimitably sardonic manner, the *Wizard of Oz* anthem "Ding Dong, the Witch Is Dead." He proceeded to declare that he would like to dance on her grave and expressed the desire to drive a stake through her heart—which is how, according to legend, one kills a vampire once and for all. Written out of her will, he reveled in the thought that she died a friendless woman. He once more recited the incidents of abuse he had experienced at her hands and described how they had tortured each other relentlessly. His greatest regret, he reported, was that he never physically assaulted her. It was at this point that Dr. Greer first proposed that perhaps Leo's father had recreated Nazi Germany within his own family and then escaped; Leo agreed that this seemed a tenable hypothesis. Finally acknowledging that he felt some twinges of sadness, Leo did admit that he had bought a mourning candle. But he emphasized that he was not sitting *shivah* for his mother and prayed for her only once a day rather than the traditional three times; he declared that he had been more upset at the death of his father several years earlier. Noting that in accord with their wishes, both of his parents had been cremated—a procedure that is prohibited in the Jewish faith—Leo observed that one of the reasons that the Holocaust was so horrific was that Jews were never supposed to be cremated. Dr. Greer suggested that perhaps Leo's parents had, even in death, identified with the Jewish victims.

Several weeks after his mother's death, Leo's phobia about vampires returned. Initially, he was not aware of it, since it was hidden behind counterphobic rituals. Leo began to speak of a ritual he had developed for the end of his sessions, which were scheduled just before lunch. At the end of each session, he would go to a deli to order what he called an "antisocial sandwich," pastrami on Lebanese bread—"antisocial" not only because of the long-running political conflict between Israel (as represented by the conventionally "Jewish" smoked meat) and Lebanon (the bread), but also because of its pungent smell of onions and garlic. As Dr. Greer reminded Leo, garlic is another conventional protection against vampires. The developing ritual suggested that the patient was anxious that his mother, like a vampire, would prove immortal by continuing to torment him. Leo could not start a normal mourning process, and his difficulty in mourning could only be observed indirectly, as in this ritual.

Another event that occurred around this time provided further indirect evidence of his inability to mourn. While following Diana to his home, Leo was pulled over by the police for speeding. After appearing at traffic court, where the judge upbraided him for speeding in a neighborhood where children and animals might wander into the street, Leo was furious with the judge, as well as with the lawyer who had represented him in court. He was also appalled that Diana had suggested that he should not have stopped, since there was only one patrol car to stop them both; Leo was in the second car and could have kept going. Diana's suggestion that he break the law suddenly made her appear to be a dangerous woman who could ruin his life. Screaming that Dr. Greer, in the name of therapeutic neutrality, was refusing to tell him whether Diana was a sociopath, Leo worried that without Dr. Greer's intervention, he might once more commit himself to a "bad" woman and get "assassinated," as he put it. Behind this outburst, Dr. Greer sensed, was unspoken guilt; in Leo's fantasies, he had "assassinated" his mother, and that guilt was impeding his bereavement process. Furthermore, his mother—"alive" in Diana as the vampire "bad woman"—could come back and kill him, he feared. During this session, Leo could not lie still on the couch and, after reporting his court appearance and his rage toward Diana, would not speak; he was paralyzed with extreme rage and anxiety. In his fantasies, he was on trial for the murder of his mother and, to prove his innocence to Dr. Greer, was denying his (oral) aggression with muteness.

In the next session, Leo reported a dream in which he had been found guilty of a crime and was placed in a cell with a huge, muscular inmate. The inmate said, "Let's play house," to which Leo replied, "Fine: I'll be papa and you be mamma." The inmate retorted, "Come here then and suck mamma's penis." Leo described the inmate as both a man and a woman and thus as "an imposter." No one, this dream seemed to suggest, seemed to be what "he" or "she" really was; a woman could have a penis, a Jew could pass as a Nazi, and so on. Leo began to laugh. The image of his "phallic mother" was tamed; it was even comical. It was in the next session that Leo finally expressed a touch of regret that he had not gone to visit his mother before her death. He also acknowledged to Dr. Greer that there was one positive quality that he got from his mother, an appreciation of the arts and culture. And he jokingly vowed not to eat any more "antisocial sandwiches"; his fear of the vampire mother had diminished, at least for a while.

Mourning and Moving On?

When Leo decided to sell his house not long after his mother's death, Dr. Greer sensed that Leo's preoccupation with the house was his way of trying to complete the mourning process for both his mother and father, albeit in an indirect manner. In Leo's associations, the house, through displacement, represented his parents, especially his "bad" mother. By selling it, Leo would learn to mourn and to separate himself from parental images.

In a dream around this time, Leo found himself in the house he had lived in with his mother and brother in early adolescence. He was doing his homework, but worried that his mother had not yet returned from her bridge game. In the dream, she did not come home at all that night, and Leo went to bed extremely anxious. When he awoke (still in the dream) the next morning, he discovered Diana in bed with him. Hearing his mother come in, he saw, as she passed his bedroom door, that she was annoyed because she had to care for him. She returned to his bedroom to attack him with a hairbrush—the brush with which, in reality, she had beaten him when he was a child. He struggled with her, and she kicked him in the groin; before the fight was over, both were injured and bleeding. Leo awoke with anxiety. While associating to the dream, Leo recalled how anxiously he had waited on the front stoop for his mother to come home during his "latch-key" years, fearing that she would never return. As an adolescent, he had once threatened his mother with a steak knife; the rest of the time, he symbolically slashed at her with caustic remarks. He also recalled how his mother regularly walked around the house in her underwear and left the bathroom door open when she used the toilet. Leo began to wonder whether his adolescent aggression toward her had not been a defense against incestuous wishes: the first time Leo had been able to touch upon the childhood psychosexual difficulties that had been hidden beneath his aggressive conflicts.

As Leo contemplated selling his house, he also expressed a wish to terminate his treatment—a transference wish to separate and individuate from the mother/analyst. Leo stated that he was afraid that Dr. Greer might hate him and wish to get revenge; instead, Dr. Greer responded by asking Leo about his difficulty in mourning the loss of his mother. Leo could not yet allow himself to feel full sadness over his mother's death, since his mother's "bad" image was still in his mind. "A leopard never changes its spots," he responded. Instead, Leo openly expressed sadness over the loss of his ex-wife. In the same session, he reported a short dream in which he performed auto-fellatio. This dream expressed his wish to be totally self-sufficient; if Leo could separate from his mother's (and Dr. Greer's) image, he would not have to depend on anyone again, nor would he be at anyone's mercy.

Selling the house was also connected with his father's image and the legacy of the Third Reich that the father had transmitted to him, as first became clear when Leo called the couple who planned to buy his house "arrogant" for refusing to include a clause in the contract to release him from responsibility for any defects found in the house after it was inspected. Dr. Greer suggested that Leo was afraid that if the house were re-inspected, the couple (Nazis) would find defects in the house (proof that he was a Jew) and would kill him. If the buyers were Nazis, he had to be careful, to control the transaction so as to assure that they would not discover any mistakes—again, like his father incognito in Nazi Germany. In the end, however, Leo sold his house to this couple.

Though the following story did not surface until later in his analysis, it seems clear in retrospect that Leo's "Nazi-fication" of the prospective buyers echoed another instance of paternal "paranoia." Soon after Leo was married for the first time, his father and stepmother moved to the city in the Southern United States where Leo and his wife lived. While helping his father to look for a home, Leo observed that his father perceived every real estate agent in the city as anti-Semitic. The father went to great lengths to avoid making his Jewish identity known. Instead of hiring a single agent, Leo's father hired 10, and gave none of them his real name. Sometimes he used gentile aliases, though Leo does not recall what they were; at other times, he divided his last name into two parts and gave one agent one half of his name and another agent the other. We presume that Leo's father perceived this Southern city as similar to Nazi Germany; as a Jew in danger, he apprehensively tried to hide his identity as he had in Germany. In his "paranoia" surrounding the Southern realtors' putative anti-Semitism, Leo's father provided yet another model of the anxious Jewish victim.

While going through a trunk in his attic before moving, Leo found his father's college diploma and an old evaluation form from the school of economics, stating that his father was a superb student and a gifted scholar. Leo also found several photographs of his father, which he now planned to have framed. Though he must have already known what was in the trunk, Leo had apparently repressed this knowledge, for he spoke of a "new" reality of his father's past. In his newfound respect for his father, Leo lamented that his father had ever married such an abusive "demon" (Leo's word) as his mother. Leo wished that his father had been able to stand up to her, still imagining his father as a cowardly man who had sacrificed his son to a vicious woman. But then Leo wondered whether his mother had sensed that her husband identified with the Nazis and had therefore become afraid of him. Had she, in turn, become identified with the Nazis herself in order to survive? "Is this what made her so hostile?" Leo reflected.

Soon after (re)evaluating his parents' images and attempting to separate from them intrapsychically, Leo began to speak of the wish to start a new life—perhaps in the western United States, where he could build his own life, raise sheep, and have children. This pastoral vision echoed not only the proverbial frontier "fresh start" of the American cultural imagination, but also the image of his father, who had gone to the western part of the country and found a "good" new wife. As Leo thought more seriously about marriage, however, he began to voice doubts about Diana. One of Leo's major concerns was that Diana would wish to have children. She had refused to convert to Judaism, which meant that in accord with Jewish tradition, their offspring would not be Jewish. The idea of having children was forbidding for Leo for other reasons as well. A relative whose mother had been a child at the time she was held captive by the Nazis told Leo that her mother had told her how the German troops used Jewish children for their sexual pleasure. For Leo, the question of having children began consciously to resonate with responsibilities to the whole Jewish people.

Leo also began to worry about Diana's fitness as a partner for him. Arriving at one session in an agitated state, he announced incredulously that Diana had failed an algebra test. He sat up on the edge of the couch, took a piece of paper out of his pocket, and jotted down the simple algebra equation that she had been unable to solve to see if Dr. Greer could solve it. Leo exclaimed that he did not want to be married to a "stupid person," nor did he want to be treated by one. To counteract this image of her as unintelligent, he had to look at her "sweet, adoring face" to melt away his aggressive fantasies about her. Nevertheless, as he later reported, he "banged" her that night, later noticing that he had another outbreak of herpes, with which he was now afraid he had infected her.

Around the same time, Leo planned to proceed with an operation to correct his reflux disease. Dreading the thought of being a patient, he arranged to have Diana stay with him while he was in the hospital to oversee the nurses; he could not trust that the doctors and nurses would not become replicas of the original objects that traumatized him as a child. After the operation, he noted, he would not be able to belch or vomit; perhaps this would stop all that "shit" that comes out of his mouth, he joked. Dr. Greer sensed both progressive and regressive aspects of Leo's preoccupation with his operation. On the regressive side, Leo was afraid to be subject to medical experimentation by dreadful doctors and nurses, who represented his "bad" Nazi mother. As a defense, he "banged" Diana and devalued her as if he were a Nazi himself. At the same time, he wished Diana to be a "good" woman, to protect him while he was in the hospital as if he were a Jewish victim. On the progressive side, finding the "strong" father (as "discovered" in the trunk in the attic) and separating from his mother's image suggested that Leo might be able to move "up" to oedipal issues, including castration anxiety. His increased castration anxiety made him fear Dr. Greer, leading Leo once more to consider ending his analysis. Before Dr. Greer could join the previous analyst in using the "amputation approach," Leo wanted to escape by terminating his analysis himself.

Interestingly, Leo underwent an endoscopic examination for his reflux disease and was told that it should be treated more conservatively. Nothing more was ever heard about his condition, and he decided to continue to work with Dr. Greer.

* * *

At the beginning of the third year of Leo's treatment, he and Diana talked about becoming engaged, provoking a major turn in Leo's analysis. Diana hesitated to discuss plans for marriage with her parents, particularly her mother, for they had already expressed their concern about the couple's differences in age and religious tradition. Based on certain innuendoes, Leo had concluded that Diana's mother was anti-Semitic and announced that neither of Diana's parents would be welcome in his new home. Leo had begun to treat Diana's parents, seemingly harmless individuals, as if they were Nazis—part of his more general pattern of using people around him to represent his own Third Reich images. They suddenly ceased to be *symbols* of anti-Semitism and actually became, in his mind, what they were supposed to represent: they became *protosymbols* (for further discussion of the relationship between symbols and protosymbols, see chapter 11). At this point Dr. Greer, through observations about Leo's transference relationship with him, showed Leo that he had been living in two worlds: one world in the present time, and the other in the period of the Third Reich. Leo, the analyst emphasized, needed both to differentiate between his two worlds and to separate symbols from protosymbols. Only then could he integrate the two worlds, achieve a more cohesive self, and establish a continuum in his psychic world.

Dr. Greer suggested that Leo resisted this integration because he wished to maintain an attachment to his existing parental representations, in spite of his felt anger against his parents' images. To acknowledge his hidden dependency on his parents might, paradoxically, help Leo to separate himself from the influence of their internalized images. For some time after this session, Leo reported a series of dreams that can be understood as "separation-individuation" (Mahler, 1968) dreams. For example, he would be sitting in restaurants with various women from his past and, in each dream, the woman would get up and leave him.

As the year progressed, Leo reported that he no longer felt so much like a "Chicken Little." Once when Diana playfully pinched him on the thigh, he reflexively responded with rage and suspicion. When he demanded to know why she behaved sadistically, she tried to assure him that she had not meant to hurt him and that she was sorry if he thought otherwise. At first, he doubted her, but then thought that if he were ever going to trust her, he had to separate her out from his abusive mother—to accept her at her word and in her own world, not automatically to regard her as a treacherous agent in a Third Reich world. He began to recognize when he was puffing himself up in response to a threat filtered through a Holocaust lens. "There I go again with the Nazi stuff," he would say.

Dr. Greer's Illness and Leo's "Escape"

As Leo made therapeutic progress, three and a half years into his treatment, Dr. Greer was diagnosed with tonsilar cancer and was told by his physician that he would have to undergo a full course of radiation, as well as a modified radical lymphectomy. Ordinarily, analysts do not disclose the details of their illnesses to their patients. However, Leo was a physician and Dr. Greer knew that he would soon see evidence of the radiation treatment. In any case, as it happened, Leo had already sensed Dr. Greer's anxiety about his illness and inquired about his health. Under these unusual circumstances, Dr. Greer decided that it would be therapeutically appropriate for him to disclose the facts about his condition to his patient. But Dr. Greer suspected how difficult it would be for Leo to express the full force of his rage in the transference now that Dr. Greer would be "unavailable."

Leo's initial response to the news was compassionate. Soon, however, Leo's anxiety reached a crescendo, and he mobilized narcissistic defenses—making plans to purchase a "most powerful" car, to travel on the Concorde, and even to reserve a seat on the first commercial flight to the moon. Soon after Dr. Greer's disclosure, Leo developed a sinus infection that required minor surgery. Whatever infectious agent caused Leo's sinus infection, it was clear that he was also identifying with his ailing therapist as a defense against the threat of separation from him. Similarly, regardless of the physical causes of Dr. Greer's cancer, his condition had evolved into a crucial psychological event between him and his patient. Leo, to allay his own anxiety, began to abuse his other doctors to his analyst. When Leo, through identification (sinus infection), saw himself as one with Dr. Greer as a "defective" person, his fear of doctors and caretakers increased—they might be Nazis.

Unfortunately, there was little time to understand and work through the psychological meaning of Dr. Greer's illness for Leo. Dr. Greer expected that Leo would experience not only unexpressed anxiety and rage at "losing" his analyst, but also a fantasy (with accompanying guilt) of having caused Dr. Greer's potentially fatal illness. Dr. Greer had no choice but to temporarily discontinue Leo's treatment because of the requirements of his own medical treatment. Leo did not want to see another therapist, and Dr. Greer assured Leo that he would resume their work together as soon as he was able.

* * *

Two months later, Dr. Greer was told by his physician that radiation therapy alone was enough to cure his cancer and that he needed no surgery. Dr. Greer's voice returned as the edema of his vocal cords subsided, and he and Leo could meet again. Leo insisted that their first session after Dr. Greer's absence be a face-to-face session. The analyst did not object, sensing that Leo needed to know that his therapist was still alive and well. Leo talked intellectually about his knowledge of tonsilar cancer. At the end of the session, Dr. Greer told Leo that in spite of the ordeal he had gone through, he felt that his analyzing faculties were intact and that he was ready to resume their therapeutic work.

Leo returned after a couple of days, lay on the couch as usual without protest, and immediately reported a dream in which he was driving a car with Diana as a passenger. In the dream, he pulled into a Burger King restaurant that resembled a 1950s diner situated beside an ocean. As he got out of his car, he noticed something dangerous and shouted to his girlfriend that they needed "to get out of there." Immediately after reporting the dream, Leo began to speak rather ramblingly on several subjects: a severe sore throat he had developed the previous night; the president of the United States, who had given a foreign policy speech; and his remorse over how badly he had treated people in the past, particularly those who did not deserve it. Leo then mentioned that this was the anniversary of his father's death and that he regretted not having been a better son. However, he continued, he simply could not tolerate the man's "craziness," even though he knew that his father was unable to control the symptoms. On the other hand, Leo proceeded, he had treated his mother more considerately than she deserved, so he had no remorse about her. But, he disclosed, he had been "conscience-stricken" since Dr. Greer's illness; he considered himself an unregenerate misanthrope.

This dream and the seemingly extraneous thoughts that followed revealed much about Leo's perception of Dr. Greer's illness. When he knew that his therapist could not take care of him, he related to Dr. Greer as an inadequate mother; the 1950s diner by the ocean signified his regression and the image of the unsafe mother who would not feed or tend him properly. But the diner also represented his father's image (Burger *King*/president). He turned to his father's image for security, but once more he was disappointed; the father was too "crazy" (anxious) to help him. Receiving no solace from the parental images played a key role in his identification with their defective images. What was missing in Leo's dream and his associations was his rage against the parental representations/Dr. Greer and the accompanying feelings of guilt. This hidden guilt was the prime motivation for Leo's shamefaced misanthropy and for his identification with the ill Dr. Greer (Leo's sore throat). By his next session, this identification became clearer. Reporting a dream in which a crab attacked his neck, Leo immediately recalled that the Latin word for "crab" was *cancer*.

Leo's thoughts suddenly turned from this dream, however, to his murderous rage against his mother and the wish that he had revenged himself on her. Leo expressed no rage directly toward Dr. Greer himself. But Leo expressed his rage against his analyst indirectly during this session by involuntarily soiling his pants while lying on the couch—an act of anal rage. Dr. Greer suggested that this accident was an oblique expression of Leo's regressive rage toward his therapist and proposed to Leo that he might unconsciously believe that his rage had caused not only his therapist's cancer, but also his mother's death. What really troubled

Leo, Dr. Greer continued, were his feelings of guilt and his fear of abandonment.

In spite of Dr. Greer's efforts to help Leo feel and work through his guilt and fear of abandonment, Leo was filled with self-reproach and depressive affect for weeks. Once more, Leo returned to his preoccupation with "fixing" Diana, with turning her into an ideal object. At this time Leo recalled an important piece of information about his infancy: that, during the first months of his life, he had been cared for by a nurse. Of course, he could not recall this nurse or how she took care of him. Nor did he know why she was the main mothering figure in the earliest part of his life: Was Leo's mother suffering from a postpartum depression that required the services of another woman to take care of Leo? Was the nurse a nurturing figure? Was there an early experience of "good" mothering followed by "bad" mothering? Though we will never know the factual answers to these questions, we can nevertheless assume that the infant Leo suffered a significant object loss when the nurse left. Although he had no formed and separated image of this nurse, it is possible that her existence explains why Leo tried to create an ideal woman image whenever he regressed in the face of perceived danger.

When Leo's various attempts to "fix" Diana frustrated him, he returned to expressing his rage through Nazi images. Leo began to revile homosexuals, another group marked for extermination under the Third Reich; verbally attacked handicapped people; and assailed psychoanalysis as a pseudo-science. Dr. Greer's illness had made him a handicapped person, and his profession had been disparaged by the Nazis. Leo would either "kill" Dr. Greer and be a guilty and abandoned person forever, or "escape," as he put it, from psychoanalysis. In spite of the analyst's efforts to help Leo to work through this unbearable dilemma, Leo broke away from treatment. Dr. Greer did not hear from Leo for a year and a half.

Returning to Therapy

About 18 months after the patient's "escape," Dr. Greer received a telephone call from Leo asking to re-enter analysis. Since he had last seen Dr. Greer, Leo said, he had not achieved a moment's peace with his conscience, so tormented was he by guilt and self-hatred for how badly he had treated others (in the transference, Dr. Greer) in the past. He had gone to a physician who gave him an antidepressant, but his self-hatred continued unabated. Dr. Greer agreed to resume Leo's treatment.

When they met, Dr. Greer reminded Leo that he might possess a fantasy that he was the cause of the therapist's cancer and that this fantasy might have impelled him to abandon his treatment. At first, Leo denied that his pangs of conscience had anything to do with Dr. Greer's cancer. Reluctantly, however, he admitted that there was indeed something that he had consciously withheld because he was concerned that it might upset the therapist. One of Leo's patients, who had been treated with radiation decades previously for tonsilar cancer, had just been diagnosed with a radiation-induced cutaneous carcinoma that would ultimately take his life. Leo suddenly realized that he had displaced his guilt over the fantasy that he had caused Dr. Greer's illness to his patient. Dr. Greer explained to Leo that he was neither as weak and helpless nor as omnipotent and destructive as Leo imagined he was. Their therapeutic work thus resumed and has continued for more than a year and a half as we prepare this book.

Leo expresses his wish—and has made successful attempts—to stop living in the world of the Third Reich. He has begun to think about being Jewish—out in the open—without much anxiety. In the fourth month after resuming therapy, Leo dreamed that hitching a ride across the country, he was picked up by a man in a truck. Suddenly realizing that he is wearing his yarmulke, Leo surreptitiously removes it, but when the two men arrive at their destination and get out of the truck, Leo notices that the driver himself is wearing a skull cap. Leo is surprised, because the man did not appear to be Jewish, and feels ashamed that he did not have the courage to wear his openly. Leo intuitively understood that the day's residue for this dream was a conversation he had had the previous evening with Diana, whom he planned to marry, about choosing the religious tradition in which they would raise their future child. As Diana expressed second thoughts about their earlier decision to follow Jewish custom in this matter, Leo still felt concerned that if they raised their children as Jews, the children might face difficulties in the "present world" in which Leo lives.

But the dream also had a transference implication: Dr. Greer (who in reality is not Jewish), as the representative of the Jewish oedipal father, would allow Leo to accept his "natural" identity as a Jew without anxiety. After discussing this dream, Leo began to (re)experience oedipal struggle with Dr. Greer, accompanied by Leo's attempts to differentiate between his "crazy" father and a "new" object, Dr. Greer. Once more the father's "paranoid schizophrenia" appeared in the treatment. Dr. Greer proposed that Leo's father was most likely not a true schizophrenic and that his symptoms represented a defensive adaptation to having been a Jew among Nazis. While struggling with this suggestion, Leo began to experience a different internal course with oedipal issues, as well as with the image of his mother. The concretized aggression and direct references to Nazi elements in his dreams and daily life began to give way to symbolic expressions of his aggression.

About a year before the preparation of this book, Leo and Diana married. As the couple began to talk seriously about starting a family, Leo's effort to go through an oedipal struggle began in earnest. As has been typical for him, he began this process with an enactment. One day Leo arrived for his appointment accompanied by Diana, who waited in the waiting room during her husband's session. Leo reported to a surprised Dr. Greer that Diana had come with him to the doctor's office because they were leaving on a trip together immediately after the session. Nevertheless, symbolically, Leo had engineered an oedipal situation: two men and one woman. For months following the event, Leo exhibited an intense oedipal transference and castration anxiety. Preoccupied with castration themes, such as losing one of his teeth, he sometimes imagined, too, that it was Dr. Greer who felt castrated. For example, Leo once detailed the story of a patient's surgery on his penis. Later he reported that as he related the story, he fantasized that Dr. Greer, sitting behind him, was anxiously crossing his own legs in fear of castration. Most interesting is the fact that when Nazi images appeared in Leo's new version of the oedipal passage, he no longer experienced them as protosymbols. For example, Leo reported that in a dream in which his left deltoid muscle had atrophied (suggesting castration), he noticed a Nazi armband on his withered left arm. But now Leo knew that the Nazi symbol was a defense against his castration anxiety. At times, Leo still deployed the defense of grandiosity against taking a dependent/submissive oedipal child position. He began to speak openly of his wish to learn how to be a man and a father, however, and made efforts to resolve his oedipal conflict for the first time with a cohesive self.

After Leo went through these processes, Diana became pregnant, reigniting Leo's anxiety about fatherhood. Two events during Diana's pregnancy particularly helped to solidify Leo's reality testing. First, a visit to England during Diana's pregnancy helped him to develop a firmer sense of himself as a parent. While abroad, Leo traced the whereabouts of two cousins who had escaped Nazi-occupied Poland as teenagers. Though they told him that they knew little about his father's work in England, they gave Leo a letter his father had written to British government officials in an effort to save Jews trapped in Nazi territories. Reading this letter helped Leo first to separate the courageous father from the "schizophrenic" one and then to be able to place them on a continuum, so that his representation of his father became continuous, rather than fragmented. Second, ultrasound confirmed that the fetus was entirely healthy and normal; soon after, Leo began to identify with Dr. Greer as a good father with whom he could identify. At times, however, Leo wondered whether Dr. Greer would be envious of him when Leo himself became a father. In a dream that is actually rather typical for a neurotic man in analysis in the midst of an oedipal transference, Leo began comparing the image of his penis and sexual power with Dr. Greer's penis and sexual power. Meanwhile, Leo's fear of fatherhood began to dissipate. In another dream, Leo is going up the stairs when he notices a fellow physician and his attractive wife coming down. As the couple passes by Leo, he notices that his colleague's wife's buttocks are not covered (we recall that as a child Leo was exposed on many occasions to his undressed mother in the bathroom). Leo brushes against this attractive woman, and she reports it to her husband. Leo suddenly senses his colleague's presence "behind me" (Dr. Greer, of course, sits behind Leo during his sessions); the colleague follows Leo to a bar, where he confronts Leo about the sexual overture to his wife. Expecting that a fight will break out between him and his colleague, Leo replies, "You don't expect me to admit to that, do you?" But his colleague says, "It is okay. Let's have a drink." The two men exchange toasts and get along famously. This dream and the patient's associations to it lead us to believe that the dream indicates Leo's wish and efforts to find a resolution to his oedipus complex. As we write, much of Leo's fear of fatherhood has dissipated, and he and his wife are eagerly awaiting their son's birth. For all practical purposes, Leo has ceased to fear that his offspring will face the fury of the Nazis.

* * *

We cannot report the final outcome of Leo's treatment, as it is ongoing, but we are quite hopeful that Leo's treatment will ultimately succeed. Leo has recently been able to give us more information concerning the transgenerational transmission of images and tasks from his father to him. He has remembered, for example, that his father would become extremely anxious that they would get lost whenever they drove into the city, and that, a small boy at the time, Leo would stand up in the well of the back seat and twirl his father's hair in an attempt to comfort the man. Among other meanings of this memory, our therapeutic focus was on his attempt to soothe his father so that his father could be a better parent to him. Later Leo internalized what passed between him and his father at these moments and became both the image of anxious father/Jewish victim and the image of himself, devoted to rescuing the victim. Because he needed to be rescued himself, however, Leo was also hateful toward this victimized father-image, identifying with the Nazis to punish the anxious father.

Leo has unrepressed another significant childhood memory that, we believe, in the context of his other recollections and enactments, suggests how Leo's father may have deposited in his son the traumatized self- and object-images that have reverberated so powerfully through Leo's life. Nightly, Leo's father would come to the child's room to say "good-night" to his son. Lovingly, by Leo's account, he would sit down with his child and run his hands through the boy's hair. But every night after this display of affection, Leo's father would pass gas while sitting on the child's bed. Leo recalls his father's strange conduct quite vividly. The gas-passing, Leo reports, was so intense that his bed would actually vibrate. We conclude that the older man's nightly "gassing" of his Jewish son provided an image of the father as a Nazi murderer and an image of Third Reich history. In conjunction with Leo's role as a reservoir of history-related images, the repetition of this behavior might have formed a source of Leo's expressions of anal rage against his mother and, later, his analyst, discussed earlier in this chapter.

Leo's case will be discussed further in the final chapter's discussion of technical issues. Meanwhile, our case studies will continue with the story of "Uta," a German woman of nomadic heritage who exhibited symptoms and character traits that reflected not only her own developmental conflicts, but also the psychological influences of her nomadic background; aspects of her internalized object relations and interpersonal relations were also refracted through the prism of what had happened to members of her large group during the Nazi period. As an adult, she was under the spell of her unconscious fantasies and internalized images of the victims and victimizers of the Third Reich era.

7

Uta

A "GYPSY" UNDER WHITE LINEN

A TALL, 26-YEAR-OLD SINGLE WOMAN, Uta began analysis after the death of her boyfriend of 8 years, representing herself to her analyst, Dr. Ast, as a middle-class, career-oriented German woman. Early in her analysis, however, her primary large-group identity began to appear much less certain than Uta had reported. While discussing her father's sporadic heavy drinking, Uta portrayed drunkenness, fights, and unemployment as routine among her paternal relatives, whom she described as living in a kind of trailer park. In the course of talking about their behavior and her relation to it, Uta declared her father's family "bad," called him a "Gypsy," and referred to herself as a "Traveler."

In present-day Germany, as in most other current contexts, the word *Gypsy* (in German, *Zigeuner*) is a derogatory term: Indeed, majority groups since the Middle Ages have used this word to denote inferiority: dirtiness, dishonesty, racial or ethnic degeneracy. In this chapter, however, we will frequently use the words *Gypsy* and *Traveler* instead of the terms that nomadic persons now use to define themselves because Uta herself—consciously or unconsciously echoing Nazi practice, as well as majority usage over the centuries—employed these terms.

Jean-Pierre Liégeois (1994), who has compiled information on such communities in Germany and elsewhere for the Council of Europe, comes to the conclusion that the communities frequently denominated as Gypsies "comprise a *mosaic of small, diverse groups*, a moving mosaic of constantly changing patterns, a kaleidoscope in which each element retains its own particularity. Thus, *no generalizations can be made* regarding the origins, history, language accommodations, characteristic trades, etc. Yet, a shared base does exist" (p. 12). Although these highly variegated nomadic communities now call themselves by their own specific names, the "shared base" that Liégeois describes encompasses the two major groups of Indo-European people in Europe: *Roma* and *Sinti*. Believed to have begun their migration from India in the 9th century, the groups' main arrival in Europe occurred between the 14th and 15th centuries. In the 18th century, linguists discovered that their common language, Romani, derived from popular dialects similar to Sanskrit. Another nomadic group that will figure in our discussion of Uta's case is the *Lalleri*, a relatively small subgroup of Indo-European people in Germany numbering about 1,000.

Travelers, in Germany as elsewhere, is a term that refers to peoples who, while also nomadic by tradition, are of an origin other than East Indian. In Germany called *Jenish* (in German, *Jenisch*), *Tinker* or *Tynker* in Ireland, and *Quinquis* in Castile, Travelers were originally indigenous nomadic groups determined not by ethnicity but by social status. During the course of the Black Death in 14th-century Europe, urban populations were devastated, and many impoverished people were forced to live in the streets. To keep the cities clean during the epidemic, laws limiting beggars, circus people, street singers, and gamblers to 3 days' stay in any city were passed in the regions that eventually become the modern state of Germany, as in many other parts of Europe. Predictably, legal intolerance quickly spawned societal intolerance of such itinerant people. Shunned by settled people as devious and unclean, these unwanted individuals began to build a solidarity among themselves (Jütte, 1988), developing a "secret" language called *Rotwelsch*—literally, "dirty speaking." *Rot* probably comes from the Dutch, and means "dirty" or "rotten"; *welsch* designates any language that is incomprehensible (Siewert, 1996). Initially, this language developed by associating new meanings with existing German words: for example, *trittling* ("stepping") became a word that meant "shoe," *Breitfuß* ("broad foot") came to stand for "goose." As Travelers traversed the continent, Rotwelsch also adopted French, Latin, Yiddish, and Hebrew words. When the Roma and Sinti arrived in middle Europe, culturally "mixed" groups were formed "as elements of Indian origin"—including Romani words—"were absorbed and reinterpreted indigenous elements" (Liégeois, 1994, p. 24). As outside investigators observe, "the line between 'Gypsies' and 'Travelers' is not always a clear one, and asking to which category a given group belongs is an irrelevant and indeed unanswerable question in some contexts: intermediary groups have been in existence for a very long time, and new ones are still forming" (Liégeois, 1994, p. 37). Since the early 18th century, German Travelers have called themselves and their language Jenish, a name derived from the Romani word *dšan* ("to know"), and meaning, among the Travelers, "witty or clever" (Pott, 1844 and 1845).

There is no indigenous written history of Roma, Sinti, and Travelers or of their languages, Romani and Rotwelsch, a fact that has itself contributed to the historical stigmatization of these groups. Over the last 500 years, some who had contact with Travelers sketched rudimentary Rotwelsch lexicons so that law officers who dealt with Travelers could understand them. But Rotwelsch thus became synonymous with *Gaunersprache*: "criminal-speak." Travelers consequently became identified with criminality to such an extent that one turn-of-the-century writer (Gross, 1899) categorically states that anyone who uses even one word of Rotwelsch is a criminal. Even one of the most-cited dictionaries of Rotwelsch, which was published in 1956, openly upholds Gross's belief (Wolf, 1956). A song sung in 1957 by a choir of the Protestant Youth at a festival in Schillingsfürst in southern Germany summarizes the centuries-old prejudice against Jenish people: If anything unusual or "bad" happens in the quiet city of Schillingsfürst—even bad weather, a flat tire, or one's own toothache or sleeplessness—it is the fault of the Travelers (who settled in the city in the 18th century); if anything is stolen, the thief is definitely a Traveler. The song makes fun of scapegoating, but at the same time, it reflects a long history of bigotry.

In present-day Germany, Travelers reject identification with Roma and Sinti peoples, despite the groups' common experience of persecution. Because both of Uta's parents were of mixed Jenish, Gypsy, and German heritage, as Dr. Ast in time would learn, it was especially significant that Uta, at the beginning of her analysis, presented her father as a "Gypsy,"with that word's thoroughly negative connotations. Since most settled Germans, unlike the migrant peoples themselves, do not differentiate between the various identities of nomadic groups, Uta presented her father's background to her German analyst in a stereotyped way. Beyond her disparaging remarks about her father's family, Uta initially showed no more curiosity about her nomadic background; only in the third year of her analysis did she become "aware" that her mother was half Jenish and half German and that her father was half Jenish and half Roma. And as time went on, she demonstrated her lack of knowledge of what had happened to itinerant peoples in Germany during the Nazi period, the era in which her parents had grown up.

Uta's parents were born in the early 1930s; her mother was 13 and her father 16 when World War II ended. Her parents' developmental environment, then, was that of Nazi Germany, an environment that was extremely perilous—indeed, often deadly—for members of nomadic groups. Though there are no confirmed statistics on how many Jenish were killed during the Nazi period, in Germany alone an estimated 25,000 out of some 40,000 Sinti and Roma were killed; most surviving Jenish are now settled in Switzerland. In Nazi-occupied Europe, an estimated 250,000 to 500,000 out of some 950,000 nomadic people were exterminated (Eiber, 1993; Rose and Weiss, 1991). When Uta began her analysis, she was unaware of any possible influence on her self-concept of the fact that her parents had been members of a persecuted group in Hitler's Germany. Her analysis, however, revealed just such an influence. Her object relations and psychosexual conflicts were infused with perceptions, conscious and unconscious fantasies, and defenses concerning her identity as a Traveler or "Gypsy," as well as with the nomadic peoples' relationship with the Nazis.

The psychoanalytic literature includes numerous case studies of children of Jewish Holocaust survivors who "weave [together] fantasies from [their] parents' post traumatic screens and their own developmental conflicts" (Auerhahn and

Laub, 1998, p. 360). Although there are detailed personal accounts of Gypsies who survived the Third Reich (Eiber, 1993; Ramati, 1986), we know of no thorough psychoanalytic investigation of how the mental representation of the Nazi past has settled in the minds of children of nomadic parents who survived Nazi Germany. In this chapter, we present Uta's internal world as it unfolded during her analysis: the first set of cumulative data over the *total* psychoanalytic treatment of an adult child of nomadic survivors of the Third Reich. Uta's case exemplifies how individual and large-group identities become inextricably intertwined.

Auerhahn and Laub (1998), writing about children of Jewish Holocaust survivors, state:

> The primal scene is a model for the manner in which children take possession of different kinds of forbidden knowledge by imbuing it with developmental issues. In addition, it becomes fused with Holocaust fantasies to create an alternative primal scene atrocity. It is in the context of Holocaust knowledge that all other knowledge, including the secret of where babies come from, is acquired. That is because infantile sexuality, stimulated by the erotic components of parental care, can become fused with aggressive Holocaust content if Holocaust affect and imagery are evoked in that relationship. (p. 372)

In Uta's case, her primal scene fantasies were influenced by aggressive components derived from having been a physically abused child, having slept in the same bedroom as her father from the age of 5 until she was 17, and other traumatic developmental experiences, but the fantasies were additionally contaminated with the legacy of the Third Reich. Uta's developmental conflicts were reflected in her main internal struggle between a wish to maintain her nomadic identity, on the one hand, and a wish to become identified with the aggressor, on the other; each of these reciprocal identities was associated with intense conflicts, so she could never settle whether she would become a victim of Nazi persecution or a Nazi persecutor. Preoccupied with attempts to deny, repair, or reverse her parents' large-group identity, which had been traumatized and altered by the Third Reich and then deposited into their daughter's self-representation, Uta regularly exhibited a conflict between her large-group identity as a German Traveler or Gypsy and her identification with settled Germans, a defensive adaptation to her environment.

Her parents had not shared their past experiences as Gypsy or Jenish people or both living under the Third Reich. In fact, her mother had once told her, "Our ancestors came from Austria. We had German passports, and we are Germans"—which in itself was a factually correct statement, but which, of course, did not tell the whole story of the family's internal psychological processes. As a child, Uta regularly visited her father's family at the trailer park, where she learned, to some extent, to speak the Rotwelsch that they spoke. In public with her sister, she used Rotwelsch when they did not wish to be understood by others; Rotwelsch was her "secret language." Thus, Uta knew and "did not know" her nomadic heritage.

Uta is not alone among her generation in Germany; many both know and do not know what happened to nomadic peoples during the Nazi regime. Among the general public, there is much denial and repression of their tragedy; many still believe that Gypsies, unlike Jews, were not systematically targeted for extermination, and that those itinerant people who were taken to the camps were criminal or antisocial individuals, guilty of individual wrongdoings. Indeed, the 1999 decision by the German government to build a central Holocaust memorial in Berlin only in honor of Jewish victims may reflect a continuing denial of what happened to Gypsies during the Third Reich. In order to understand Uta's internal world, however, we must have a more complete and accurate grasp of the specific experience of the nomadic population in Nazi Germany.

Gypsies Under the Nazis

It is, of course, beyond our purpose to review in detail the whole history of the European Gypsies or even the complete history of nomadic peoples in Germany; suffice to say that anti-Gypsy feeling has existed for centuries in Europe. Citing the historical European conviction that blackness denotes inferiority and evil, Kenrick and Puxon (1995) suggest that Gypsies' dark skin relegated them to inferior status, noting that monk Cornerius of Lübeck wrote in 1417 that Gypsies' faces were ugly and black like those of the Tartars. Furthermore, write Kenrick and Puxon,

> Another strong factor in the unfavorable attitude in western and central Europe was the suspicion attached to anyone who crossed from the Turkish-occupied lands. [Gypsies had to travel through the Ottoman Empire to find their way to Europe from India.] From that direction came infidels, enemies of religious states and the church. Lacking an organized religion of their own, the Gypsy were [sic] from the beginning open to attack by Christian and indeed Muslim clergy. (Kenrick and Puxon, 1995, p. 10)

Over time, this association of Gypsies with the Muslim "infidel" engendered the myth that the nomadic peoples had been cursed by God because they had refused shelter in their tents to Joseph and Mary on their flight from Egypt (Kenrick and Puxon, 1995). In 1749, a huge round-up of Gypsies in Spain was based on their purported threat to Christianity and alleged practice of cannibalism. In Hungary in 1782, 200 nomadic persons were tried and tortured until they confessed to being cannibals. These are only a very few of the incidents of persecution to which itinerant peoples have been subjected over many centuries on the pretext that they are an ungovernable people, given to perverse and subversive behavior.

In fin de siècle Germany, a Gypsy Information Bureau (Zigeuner-Nachrichten Dienst) was opened in Munich on the grounds that Gypsies constituted "a 'plague' (*Zigeunerplage*) from which the public must be protected through vigilant surveillance" (Liégeois, 1994, p. 131). Among the many bureaucratic paradoxes to which nomadic communities were subject was the demand for fixed domicile from persons who were, at the same time, forbidden to build houses. Anti-Gypsy sentiment was especially virulent in Bavaria, where laws enacted in 1928 placed all nomadic peoples under constant police surveillance (Liégeois, 1994).

By the time the Third Reich came to power, then, German ground was already deeply sown with anti-Gypsy sentiment. As early as 1933, the Race and Settlement Office (Rasse- und Siedlungsamt) of the SS in Berlin demanded that Gypsies and half-Gypsies be sterilized. In 1934, various agencies of the Nazi Party attempted to exclude Gypsies from professional organizations. In 1936, Heinrich Himmler, the newly appointed chief of the German Police, ordered the centralization of criminal police activities, making the surveillance and control of nomadic peoples easier than ever before. In the same year, the Race Hygiene and Population Biology Research Center, linked to the German National Health Office, was established under the directorship of Dr. Robert Ritter, whose racist views on Gypsies, part-Gypsies, and Jenish are well documented (Ritter, 1937, 1938, 1939, 1940–1941). Preoccupied with eliminating such objectionable peoples from a National Socialist Germany, he recommended that any sexual contact between Gypsies and ethnic Germans be legally proscribed, that any future reproduction of these "undesirables" be prevented finally and forever, and that all Gypsies be detained in the forced labor camps established in the 1930s, fenced by barbed wire and kept under constant SS or police surveillance. In addition, Ritter supported similar studies and enforced sterilization of "antisocial families," by which he clearly means Jenish people.

The Nazi preoccupation with "pure Gypsy blood" (as, indeed, their preoccupation with racial "purity" more generally) is in large part derived from 19th-century ethnological and philological studies, which demonstrated that many languages and language groups used from Europe to India—including Sanskrit, Zend, Persian, Greek, Latin, Celtic, Teutonic, and Slavonic, with their modern representatives—share a common root. This shared source of the Indo-European languages, designated by the term *Arian*, ran the theory, had originated from the Baltic area. From there, people using this language spread south as far as the areas occupied by the modern nations of Iran and India. The first known use of the name "Arian" for these peoples appears in documents dating to 1000 B.C.E. which describe Arians' clashes with the indigenous populations in these areas, which eventually absorbed the newcomers' language. About 2,000 years later, some Arian groups moved westward, where they were called Tsigeuner (German, *Zigeuner*, "the untouchable ones"): "Gypsies." Because Hebrew does not belong to the group of Indo-European languages, it must have been easy for the Nazis to characterize the Jews as an impediment to the effort to create a "pure Aryan race." The Gypsies, however, had migrated from locations where the original Arians had lived and spoke an Arian language. Thus, Hitler and the National Socialist "scientists" became preoccupied with determining who was a "pure Gypsy," so that such individuals could be relocated to special areas to be studied further. Behind such an idea, we believe, might have been an attempt to "re-breed" pure Aryans, just as one would re-breed a "pure blood" animal in a zoo. Accordingly, the most dangerous group was considered to be composed of those who were part-Gypsy and part-German, as the Jenish were—and a person with as little as one-eighth "Gypsy blood" counted as a part-Gypsy. Only by preventing the continued procreation of the mixed population, Ritter advised, would future generations of Germans be free of this "scourge."

Beginning in 1936, everyone who did not fit the National Socialist standard began to be taken to camps. Because the nomadic population was not homogeneous, and because many Gypsies and Travelers often moved from one location to another, the Nazis had a more difficult time identifying Gypsies than isolating Jews, whose names and religion were often recorded in many official documents. It was in 1938 that the combined efforts of the criminal police and the racial "scientists" produced Himmler's "Basic Decree" on "The Fight Against the Gypsy Menace": "This is to 'begin settlement of the gypsy question with regard to the existence of the race'" (Rose and Weiss, 1991, p. 188). Gypsies as a group were categorized "scientifically" by Nazi "experts," but the final decision to classify an individual as Gypsy, part-Gypsy, or non-Gypsy vagrant was to be made by the criminal police on the advice of specialists. Regardless of the official decision, however, every individual under suspicion of being a Gypsy had to be registered by fingerprints and photographs with the criminal police from the age of 6, and all were forced to undergo biological measurements and examinations by racial "experts," according to protocols developed by Dr. Ritter.

It appears that Himmler initially wished to preserve two groups as "museum pieces": those who were "pure" Sinti or "pure" Lalleri. But Himmler's plans, perverse as they were, were overruled by other Nazi authorities, such as Joseph Goebbels, who were of the opinion that all nomads should be exterminated without any distinction between groups. Further, the racial "scientists" determined, no pure Sinti or Lalleri existed. Nevertheless, during the escalation of the war and the evolution of the death camps in the 1940s, the Nazis continued to be obsessively preoccupied with the classification of Gypsies and of those living like Gypsies, on the basis of how much "German blood" could be determined to exist in each individual. In 1941, a refinement in Nazi racial "science" resulted in a new system of seven categories, in which some categories were considered "safer" than others. Still, because the police and racial "experts" assigned classifications, any person with a nomadic background or who was considered asocial or work-shy was in danger.

In 1936, the now-infamous Dachau camp became among the first to hold German—and, later, Austrian—Gypsies on the grounds that they were "antisocials." In December 1942, Himmler signed the "Auschwitz Decree" ordering the dispatch of all Gypsies in Germany and German-occupied lands in Europe to Auschwitz, in the south of Poland; 10,000 nomadic persons from Reich territory and another 22,000 from other parts of Europe were eventually imprisoned in the Auschwitz-Birkenau death camp. Technically, this decree exempted some subgroups: pure Sintis and Lalleris; Gypsies married to Germans; socially assimilated Gypsies with settled work and accommodations; and foreign citizens. But when "the police rounded up Gypsies they in fact took little notice of these exceptions" (Kenrick and Puxon, 1995, p. 43). Again, it is clear that all nomadic persons and individuals with nomadic large-group identities, regardless of the obsessive official classifications, were endangered. All were considered asocial and criminal.

Ludwig Eiber's 1993 account of the persecution of Sinti and Roma in Munich from 1933 to 1945, *Ich wusste, es wird schlimm* ("I Knew It Would Become Awful"), reveals that Nazi behavior toward these groups was different in some ways from the regime's treatment of Jews. For example, Gypsies were permitted to live as families and were assigned to quarters in Auschwitz that were separate from the areas where Jews were located. While Jews were considered infectious invaders into the German body, the Nazis viewed Gypsies as more fully human. Nevertheless, they were considered to be lower human beings (*Untermenschen*): congenitally antisocial, criminal, alcoholic, and dirty, associated with human waste. Their moral and biological development was thought of as unrefined, unstructured, and uncontrolled. To the Nazis, nomadic peoples were a promiscuous horde who freely indulged incestuous and other perverse impulses.

It can be argued that whereas Jews, in general, were subjected to an "instantaneous" genocide after 1941, nomadic peoples, in general, were subjected to a slowed-down, drawn-out one—though, eventually, this "differentiated" system for fighting the "enemies of German blood" did break down. It is certainly well documented that like Jews, nomadic persons were gassed and murdered; Josef Mengele's first act upon becoming an SS camp doctor in Auschwitz in 1943 was to order several hundred Sinti and Roma to the gas chambers. Nevertheless, in general, Gypsies were to be "allowed" to live and work as long as they could not procreate. While they, like Jews, were subjected to various "medical experiments," starvation, and death by labor and bad hygienic conditions, sterilization was one of the first measures suggested for the control of the nomadic peoples. Indeed, it became the principal means adopted for their prolonged genocide, though eventually its use was not confined to nomadic groups. Individuals who were deemed mentally defective or prone to develop certain diseases considered genetically transmitted were also included among those subjected to sterilization; as part of "medical experiments," some Jews were also sterilized.

The Nazis tested a number of different methods of sterilization in the effort to find "a cheap, quick method which could be used for the mass sterilization of women who were regarded by the National Socialists as racially or socially inferior" (Fings, Heuss, and Sparing, 1997, p. 92). One method of sterilization often used was to inject silver nitrate into the fallopian tubes and uterus through the genitalia; X rays of the woman's abdomen were then taken to confirm that the uterus was sufficiently destroyed to ensure infertility (Eiber, 1993). This procedure was very painful—and potentially deadly, if the silver nitrate entered the peritoneal cavity.

Sterilization of "undesirables" also took place outside of camps. For example, "Gypsy women married to Germans were operated on . . . in widely separated places and at different periods" (Kenrick and Puxon, 1995, p. 148). To be a Gypsy, to be considered Gypsy-like, or to be a socially unacceptable woman of child-bearing age, then, was like having Damocles' sword hanging over one's head during those terrible years. When a young nomadic woman reached age 14, she became subject to the threat of forced sterilization. If an "undesirable" woman "freely" subjected herself to sterilization, the Nazis promised freedom in turn. In spite of this promise, however, it is now well-known that a majority of the Gypsy population in Germany and Nazi-occupied areas of Europe was eventually killed without mercy.

Further, until the early 1960s, a wide circle of German society, including the political establishment, did not consider the mistreatment and murder of nomadic people a Nazi crime. Indeed, "In 1947 Dr. Robert Ritter became the Chief Youth Physician in the municipal health office of the city of Frankfurt-on-Main" (Margalit, 1997, 1, p. 110), reflecting the continuing acceptability of his views on the "Gypsy character." Only in 1985 did West Germany officially recognize responsibility for the persecution and extermination of nomadic peoples.

At the turn of the millennium, there remains a "Gypsy problem" in Europe. After World War II, governments across Europe made efforts—with varying degrees of "success"—to settle the nomadic population and to find permanent work for it. After the fall of the communist regimes in Eastern Europe, the increased circulation of nomadic peoples in Western Europe revived widespread prejudice. Scottish Travelers have recently reported routine harassment by the police and regular discrimination at the hands of Britain's national health service. During the 1999 war in Kosovo, Serbs forced about 100,000 Gypsies from their homes, killing hundreds. In the Czech town of Usti nad Labem, a 6-foot-high wall was built in 1999 to separate a Gypsy neighborhood from one of ethnic Czechs—an event that made the news across Europe. Those in the European Union administration working on the problem of xenophobia and racism consider the anti-Gypsy prejudice in Europe, including the Czech Republic, a major issue.

* * *

Less dehumanized than the Jews, but consistently perceived as *Untermenschen* by the majority population in Germany even before the Third Reich, Gypsies and Travelers may well have internalized some of the characteristics that were assigned to their images. Like a child who identifies not only with his parents' images, but also with the way the parents unconsciously or consciously experience the child, a suppressed minority group may identify with the image the majority group has of it (Volkan, 1999a, 1999b). In the minds of those in the German majority, to be a nomadic person was to have a primitive, uncivilized nature; the oppressed nomadic peoples' own ways of living and behaving were most likely contaminated by the majority's bigoted devaluation of the cultures of nomadic groups and racist expectation of criminal behavior and moral depravity among their members.

Uta's Personal History

Uta was born in a small, conservative German town close to Frankfurt, where, at the time of her birth, her mother was a manual worker in a shoe factory. Her father worked as a laborer in various food processing companies whenever jobs were available. In his late 40s, when Uta was 10 years old, he retired after suffering a heart attack. Uta's father's surname clearly identified his family as Gypsies in the eyes of the settled German population. Uta did not know how her parents had survived the Nazi period, though her mother had hinted that the family had passed as non-Gypsy/non-Traveler. Indeed, all of Uta's information about her parents' lives before she was old enough to observe them herself was rather sparse.

Married to a non-Traveler German who was a railroad conductor in a small town near Frankfurt, Uta's Traveler maternal grandmother had given birth to 13 children, of whom Uta's mother and her mother's elder sister were the oldest. Because nomadic people were not allowed to go to school during this time, Uta's mother barely knows how to read and write; Uta's father was also functionally illiterate. At the age of 6, Uta's mother went to work on a German farm from which she would return to her home each night. It is not clear if her "home" was in a slave labor camp for nomadic persons; Uta's mother would not reveal direct information about this question. Nevertheless, she recalled how, as a small child, she would look from a window of their "home" and see a light in a distant house. Where she lived, it seems, there was no light at night; she described the distant light as providing her an orientation in time and space. To this day, Uta's mother gazes at lights in the houses in her neighborhood before going to sleep.

At the end of the war, when she was 13, Uta's mother began to work on another German-owned farm, where she slept with the animals in the barn; she recalled "learning to speak with the animals." At this time, Uta's mother's parents were separated, leaving the abandoned wife with many young children to raise. To help her beleaguered mother, Uta's mother often brought food from the farm to her younger siblings; in fact, from 1945 on, Uta's mother essentially fended for herself. In 1950, Uta's mother married Uta's father, who was three years older. It was around this time that she became obsessed with cleanliness. So ashamed of being called a Gypsy as a child, she decided that her children should never experience such shame.

When she began her analysis, Uta had even less information about her father's side of the family before his marriage to her mother. Originally, Uta's father was married to her mother's older sister, and the couple had had one child. When the child was 3 years old, his mother (Uta's aunt) was killed in a motorcycle accident after a party. The motorcycle was driven by one of the father's brothers. Uta's mother always felt that she was not as attractive as her sister and was aware of disliking her older sibling. Despite disliking her sister's husband, too, Uta's mother assented to her own mother's wish that she marry him in order to raise the couple's child, her nephew. Uta's parents were married for 13 years before she was born. In addition to her half-brother, Uta has another brother who is some years older, and a sister who is 2 years younger.

As an adult, Uta's mother's disposition was diametrically opposed to that of her deceased older sister. She, unlike her sister, did not smoke and never missed a day at work, proving that she was not "work-shy"; we may imagine that Uta's mother was trying to identify with her German father's proletarian background. Her sister, on the other hand, appears to have identified with the more stereotypical Gypsy lifestyle, characterized by gaiety and pleasure. Her life was filled with music, dancing, laughter, and alcohol, and she was apparently unconcerned about the majority group's opinion of her. In Uta's mother's mind, as Uta would later perceive, her sister was the stereotype of the dissolute, uncivilized nomad.

As far back as Uta could recall, her mother ironed constantly, and Uta felt that the activity brought her mother comfort. In their home, the beds, couch, armchairs, and other furniture were regularly covered with freshly washed and ironed linen. It was practically unimaginable that a family member might remove the linen in order to use the furniture. Ironed and folded linen often covered the floor as well, making it difficult to walk freely in the house. When Uta was a teenager, her mother developed another obsession: Every evening she had to drink a certain brand of tea. Uta's impression was that this tea was actually necessary to her mother's life; 15 years later, Uta would learn that her mother used this tea as a laxative. If they ran out of tea, which happened often, a "disaster" would occur, forcing either Uta or her father to scour area pharmacies to replenish the depleted supply. There was a shower in the house, but Uta was never allowed to use it because her mother was concerned that she would leave water spots on the floor and walls; Uta was forced to wash herself with a wet towel in front of a sink.

There were only two rooms in the house that were not subjected to her mother's oddly fastidious treatment. The first of these was the bedroom where Uta, her father, and her younger sister had slept (in separate beds) since Uta was 5 years old—an arrangement initiated by Uta's mother after her favorite brother (Uta's uncle) was killed by his wife's lover. The wife was Uta's father's sister, who was assumed to have played a role in arranging the murder. Uta's mother may well have developed the idea that her husband's family was deadly to her family, because both her sister's and her brother's deaths were directly or indirectly caused by its members. For reasons of which we cannot be certain, however, Uta's mother began to sleep alone in the conjugal bed and exiled her husband to the next room, where Uta and her younger sister slept (Uta's childhood memory about where her brother and half-sibling slept is hazy). The door between the two rooms was kept open. With these sleeping arrangements, it is not surprising that during her analysis Uta recalled "bumping noises" (primal scene activities) and a fear that a wild man would come out of the closet during her childhood. This arrangement continued until Uta left home at the age of 17.

The other room not covered with white linen was on the second floor of the house, and it was most peculiar indeed. As a child, Uta recalled periodically becoming curious about this room—which, strangely enough, belonged to a gray parrot that was allowed to fly around the room freely, to tear the wall paper, and to defecate everywhere. Uta's mother checked on the bird frequently and spoke to it as if it were human. Always heated to harmonize with the bird's bodily needs, the room also contained a radio, which played constantly; when Uta asked to turn down the radio in the parrot's room, her mother would not allow her to do so. The room's door was left open, but the bird was trained never to fly downstairs.

Uta possessed few childhood memories about her father's side of the family. She remembered her paternal grandmother. The grandmother came to the house regularly to pick up her son to go drinking, dancing, and singing, and Uta knew that he had enjoyed such activities with his first wife. At such times, Uta recalled, her father would play the accordion. Every weekend, Uta's father took her and her sister to the home of one of his brothers—a place that, she recalled, smelled bad, but where there was freedom to play and sing without needing to be extremely cautious about the linen. Uta was even allowed to sit on the couch in the living room of her uncle's house, something she was never allowed to do in her own home. Although Uta felt free in her uncle's home, she was still careful not to stain her dress because, if she did, she knew her mother would be disgusted and beat her severely when she returned home. Uta's mother, who liked neither her mother-in-law nor the "freedom" permitted on her husband's side of the family, seldom accompanied her daughters and their father to the brother-in-law's house.

Uta's mother dressed her as if she were a princess. She often had her daughters' photographs taken in their clean and pretty dresses, and the pictures were hung on the walls of the family home. In elementary and secondary school, Uta seemed to have been an attractively dressed, comely schoolgirl. Nevertheless, she felt she was an outsider. Early in her life, Uta reported, she sensed a "madness" in her childhood environment and felt that she possessed a portion of this madness. For example, while still in kindergarten, she once climbed up on the fence along a bridge and balanced herself there in the conviction that nothing would happen to her. Furthermore, a male cousin, who lived in a trailer and who was the same age, as well as in the same class, as Uta, behaved and dressed "badly." Even as an adult, Uta considered him a typical Traveler.

On the weekends, Uta continued to go to the trailer park with her father until, ashamed to visit her Gypsy relatives, she stopped doing so during her teen years. Her awareness of something shameful within herself, however, had begun when she was 10 years old. During her analysis, she connected that feeling of shame to an incident that had taken place at that age: She was asked to take care of a baby who was sleeping in a carriage, and she shook the baby and made him cry. Uta felt that this was the most shameful thing she had ever done. It is likely, though, that the baby in the carriage was a displaced image of a physically abused Uta. As a child, she was regularly beaten by her mother, as well as by her brother and half-brother, whom her mother allowed to beat her as long as they did not hit her on her head. If the incident with the baby did, in fact, take place in reality, it might reflect an attempt to do something aggressive to another through identification with her mother and brothers; her feelings of shame might then disguise a murderous rage. Whatever the reason, Uta's sense of shame appeared openly in her prepubertal years. From an early age on, Uta had taken the responsibility of being the prime person in the family to interact with the non-Traveler environment when necessary. It was Uta who was regularly sent to the supermarket to buy food for the family. Although she enjoyed the responsibility, it also subjected her to sexual advances, unfulfillable desires, and periodic humiliation. When, for example, she tried to withdraw money from the family account only to be told there were no funds, she experienced much shame. In adolescence, Uta developed the belief that she could not have a child because she would transmit "nothing but 'bad things,'" as she said, to the child.

Uta was the first person in her family to finish any school at all. After middle school, she took up work that carried her to various countries in Europe to sell certain goods; in a sense, she was traveling like a "traditional" Jenish person, but for professional reasons. At the age of 18, she met the drug-addicted son of the wealthy family who owned the company where Uta worked as a salesperson. The affair with Bryan lasted, on and off, for 6 years before Bryan developed melanoma. When she realized that he was going to die, however, she became completely loyal to him. During the last months of his life, Bryan settled in his parents' house to die. His parents acquiesced to his wish for her to move into the house, and she took turns with Bryan's family members in caring for him. Bryan said that he wanted to marry Uta, who secretly nursed fantasies of inheriting his wealth, but the marriage never took place. After his death, Uta found herself unable to experience sadness. When Bryan's family cut off all contact with Uta, she became more aware than ever of her wish to inherit Bryan's wealth. She became preoccupied with this unfulfilled wish, of which she was deeply ashamed and which prompted her decision to seek psychoanalytic treatment. She moved to the city where Dr. Ast works, changed her profession, assumed a new post that did not require her to travel extensively, and began analysis with Dr. Ast, attending her sessions regularly three times a week.

The Initial Phase of Uta's Analysis

Images of death and destruction preoccupied Uta in the first months of her analysis—not especially unusual for a person who has experienced a loss through death as recently as Uta had. In part, Uta's preoccupation with dead people seemed to reflect an attempt, as an aspect of the work of mourning, to become identified with Bryan's image. Looking back on her work with Uta, though, Dr. Ast recalls how difficult it was for her, during the initial months of Uta's analysis, simply to understand what her patient was reporting. To Dr. Ast, Uta seemed to hide in a fog; Uta even wondered aloud whether she belonged to the generation of the dead. It would take some time for Dr. Ast and Uta to understand that the meaning of this peculiar question and of her apparent desire to identify with Bryan's image were related to Gypsy experiences during the Third Reich.

Though she professed to have been in love with Bryan, Uta pursued a promiscuous sex life until his cancer diagnosis, compulsively keeping mental lists of all her 50 or so lovers (many of whom she never met a second time) and the many locations where she had had sex. Every man with whom she had had intercourse—including Bryan, with whom her sexual activity was infrequent—was assigned a number on her list. Some of her lovers treated her badly and even abused her. Initially, it seemed to Dr. Ast that Uta wanted, in her sexual relationships, to attach herself to "clean," non-nomadic men, but her segregation of such men from "bad" Gypsy or Traveler types was not fully possible, for many of her lovers also exhibited "unwanted" elements. Bryan, in particular, was a drug addict. Uta wanted him to be completely cured and "clean" and explained her "need" to have sex with others as an attempt to make Bryan jealous enough to give up his addiction. Finally, Dr. Ast came to understand that the symbolic meaning Uta attached to Bryan's skin cancer correlated to this dialectic of cleanliness and dirtiness. Like the dirty spots Uta feared might cling to her dress when she visited her uncle's home as a young child, making her "bad" in her mother's eyes, Bryan's melanoma was like a "black spot" contaminating him, making him "bad."

Thus Uta seemed to identify with her mother's obsessional way of keeping "clean" (good) and "dirty" (bad) elements separated, an expression of anxiety about her large-group identity as a Gypsy. When she married Uta's father, Uta's mother was determined to be different from her older sister: the sister was the "Gypsy," and Uta's mother the "German." Her sister was messy, but she was clean. Thus she had carefully and absolutely separated her "clean" rooms from her "dirty" rooms; the gray bird's room appeared to represent her sister and her Gypsiness tamed and contained. In her mother's mind, Uta needed to be a clean, desirable person, but *au fond*, Uta also stood for the mother's sister and that woman's stereotyped Gypsiness. Relating to Uta with ambivalence, Uta's mother dressed her in clean clothes, but feared her daughter's dress's contamination with black spots—symbols of "bad Gypsy dirtiness." By drinking the laxative tea, the mother hoped to get rid of her own "black spots" (feces), her own "real Gypsy" coloring: an anal model of how to discard "bad" things. Relating to her mother and her image with ambivalence, Uta, too, had anal problems. When she began analysis, one of Uta's symptoms was difficulty in moving her bowels; she would sit on the toilet up to 15 minutes, shaking her body in a peculiar way, before excreting her feces.

Though this oscillation of symbolic Gypsiness and Germanness appeared in Uta's behavior patterns, she seldom referred explicitly to her nomadic background early in her analysis. Such references, however, appeared indirectly in Uta's transference reaction toward Dr. Ast. When she remarked that coming to her sessions was like doing ironing, Uta suggested that Dr. Ast's office was the location where one compulsively irons linens, folds them, and creates a clean environment. Dr. Ast sensed that Uta wished that her analyst would make her a "clean German." But such a wish was also conflicted, as became evident when Uta reported a fear that analysis would cost her the ability to laugh. Uta's mother hated to hear her daughter laugh, for laughter was characteristic of a stereotypical nomadic person.

Uta reported feeling extremely frustrated that she had not been able to see Bryan die. She had made all kinds of mental and physical preparations to be present at the moment of Bryan's death and had left specific instructions to be called if he took a turn for the worse. But his family members had failed to call her; when Uta later asked them why she had not been called, they told her that there had been no room for her in Bryan's already crowded bedroom and promptly cut off all association with Uta. Bryan was buried in a private walled cemetery, and his grave had no physical marker. After Bryan's death, she desperately wished that her mother would come to be with her in her sorrow, but "only [her] father," as she said, came to console her. In emphasizing her frustration, Dr. Ast came to believe, Uta was expressing a conflict about her status as a "replacement child." Uta was describing a strong wish, perhaps even a need, to discard the deposited elements within her, to save herself from the burden of being a replacement child.

By marrying her sister's widower, Uta's mother had replaced the dead sister in the marital bed, and thus wanted to "kill" the other woman's mental representation. In compensation for this guilty wish, the mother had kept her sister's representation "alive," to be deposited into Uta's self-representation as she had done with the gray parrot. Uta's mother used to refer to her sister as *Lebedame* (literally, "alive lady"), an unflattering epithet for someone who is sexually free and drinks, laughs, and enjoys life. Two weeks after starting her analysis, Uta partially became, in her free time, a *Lebedame*, and she stayed such for the next two years or so. She found a new boyfriend, a sculptor with whom she drank, laughed, and started having sex again, while functioning almost perfectly at work. During her analytic sessions and at work, she was a "perfect German." But she kept her life of pleasure secret from her mother. Dr. Ast sensed that if Uta could be sure that death was real, she could "kill" her mother's dead sister's representation in her and be free of living a "double life."

For about two years, Uta often experienced severe chest pain during her sessions; she would, in fact, double over with pain and get into the fetal position on the couch. During this period, Uta did not suffer these "waves" of pain outside her sessions, except on a few occasions while defecating, and she repeatedly told Dr. Ast how grateful she was that the analyst did not interfere while she was in physical pain. Uta's associations to this pain, besides references to Bryan's painful illness, were related to images of violence and danger in her childhood environment—of the parental and sibling abuse mentioned previously. Slowly, other meanings for Uta's physical misery surfaced as she and Dr. Ast began to construct Uta's unconscious fantasy of repairing the representation of her mother. First, Uta began to sense that she had caused emotional pain to her mother simply by being born; she recalled hearing that her mother had attempted suicide while pregnant with Uta. Because her mother was an unhappy, depressed, and angry woman when Uta was young, Uta had developed an unconscious fantasy of repairing and saving her mother. Uta, already a reservoir for her mother's image of her dead sister, had allowed herself to become a reservoir for her depressed and angry mother, too, assuming her mother's emotional pain and extreme aggression and expressing them as physical pain. In her transference relationship with Dr. Ast, doubling up with extreme discomfort was a way of freeing her analyst/mother from "depression" and thus creating a better analyst/mother—hence her gratitude to Dr. Ast for "allowing" her to be miserable on the couch.

Dr. Ast then understood more clearly why Bryan's death from skin cancer had so devastated and preoccupied Uta. From her childhood on, she had believed that if she were a reservoir of all "bad" things and aggression, her "partner" (mother/Bryan/analyst) would remain clean and good, giving her hope for a future nurturing relationship with that "purified" partner. Indeed, Uta had initially experienced Bryan as her depressed/unavailable mother. In reality, Bryan had been a kind man, but when he drugged himself, he would emotionally withdraw. For this reason, before Bryan contracted cancer, Uta acted like a stereotypically licentious Gypsy woman: In order to collect "badness" in herself, as if when she herself was "bad," Bryan would become "good." When Bryan developed his deadly "black spots," this change did not fit into the unconscious fantasy of repairing her partner and the corollary hope for a future good relationship. When Bryan became irreversibly "bad," she could not accept his offer of marriage and, in fact, wanted to "kill" him. Unable to create a good maternal object in Bryan, she wanted to see him die. Furthermore, with the onset of his "black spots" ("Gypsiness"), Bryan ceased to represent Uta's wished-for "good" mother and turned into the image of a dangerous, dirty Gypsy father; though Uta wanted him as an oedipal child wants her father, she was also afraid of him and wanted him "dead." For all these death wishes, however, she felt guilty, and she invested time and money in taking care of him as part of her reaction formation. When, as time went on, Uta reported regular constipation, Dr. Ast came to see that she was experiencing a complicated mourning process because she could not deal effectively with the introjected image of a "bad" (dirty, fecal) Bryan—who, in reality, had also experienced severe pains before his death. Unable to move her bowels, she kept the "bad" images within herself. The tea that Uta's mother had used to eliminate her feces (her "badness") was not working for Uta.

By the beginning of their third year of work together, Dr. Ast could clearly interpret these meanings of Uta's painful experiences and tell her patient that there might be ways for a child to relate to a depressed and angry mother other than internalizing the mother's negative qualities. She also told Uta that she need not experience such a mother in her intimate relationships with others, as if she had no other choice than to repeat the unhappy past. To help Uta differentiate Dr. Ast from the image of the mother, the analyst told Uta that she could consider her analyst to be neither depressed nor in need of being saved and repaired. Soon afterward, however, Uta reported an experience that, to Dr. Ast, reflected Uta's desire to bring to life in actions how she suffered internally to help, to repair, the other. Helping the sculptor to move his furniture to a new location, she took no breaks from the work, though some pieces were very heavy. Uta was illustrating in action how she had been a reservoir of her "bad" depressed mother/analyst's image; she did not know how to stop carrying her burden. Accordingly, Dr. Ast asked Uta what would have happened if she had taken a break from carrying the heavy furniture. In response, Uta experienced a daydream in which she was sitting down someplace relaxing and having a cigarette. In the middle of reporting her daydream, Uta reacted as if something had struck her and she stayed paralyzed on the couch for about 10 minutes, during which Dr. Ast remained silent and did not interfere. When she was able to talk again, Uta spoke of having had a visual image of a ghost leaving her body. She was paralyzed with fear that the ghost's departure from her body might kill her.

"Playing" with a Ghost

For the next 4 months, this ghost's image was "present" during Uta's sessions. As Dr. Ast and Uta "played" with the image of the ghost, it became clear that the ghost initially stood primarily for the suicidal mother and her images of the dead sister and brother, which had been deposited in young Uta's self-representation. The ghost represented, too, nomadic people generally, including Uta's own Gypsy side. Until this point, Uta was unaware of how the "Aryan versus Gypsy" issue had been condensed in her early object-relations conflicts and identifications. With the image of the ghost, however, the mental representation of the Third Reich entered openly into her analysis. Gradually, it would become clear that her early object relations and psychosexual and aggressive fantasies were deeply imbued with mental representations of Third Reich images.

Uta described the ghost as an entity with a very ugly face and big nose, but also as a victim. It occurred to her that she had seen the face depicted in a school history book reproduction of an illustration from *Der Stürmer* magazine. Published for propaganda purposes during the Nazi period, the magazine caricatured Jews as disgustingly unattractive, with big noses and oversized lips. For years, Uta had stood in front of a mirror gazing at her own face, thinking her nose big and ugly; in fact, she had often considered seeing a plastic surgeon to alter its appearance. She now knew that in her mind, to have a big nose was also to be a Nazi victim. At other times, Uta would respond to the ghost as her aggressive, abusive mother, demanding that the ghost serve her for the rest of her life. In one daydream, the ghost tried to escape as if it were a thief (a "Gypsy"), and Uta grabbed him by the nape of the neck, not allowing him to get away so easily. Thus Uta identified both as the Jewish/Gypsy victim and as the Nazi victimizer.

Uta's ghost absorbed images of her suicidal mother, her mother's sister, and Holocaust victims, but the male ghost also represented an attempt to recall fantasies about her father's penis. Uta had most likely witnessed parental intercourse as a child, which may account for the strong auditory sensations linked to her primal scene fantasies. Though the father's presence in Uta's room during her developmental years and beyond may have stimulated his daughter's oedipal strivings, Uta also saw her father as perverse and aggressive. Though she did not consciously remember having seen her parents make love, she reported "memories" of a dog sleeping in her father's bed and fantasies of her father having intercourse with this dog. Such "memories" represented her father as a stereotypically perverse and dangerous Gypsy man and herself as an incestuous oedipal dog. It seemed to Dr. Ast that Uta's perception of a perverse, aggressive father in her primal scene and oedipal fantasies was condensed with images of the aggressive brothers who had beaten her up on many occasions, for Uta could only recall one occasion on which her father had corporally punished her—and that time with a package of spaghetti. In fact, he was a kind man toward his daughters. Nevertheless, Uta wondered if her father had ever touched her sexually when he was drunk, though she was unable to recall any such incident. It is interesting to note that just before her ghost first appeared in her session, Uta had indirectly referred to this issue. After she had finished helping the sculptor with his heavy furniture, he had wanted to make love to her. When he touched her genitals, however, she suddenly had a vision of her father's hands, as if her father were touching her. Unsurprisingly, she had refused to have sex with the sculptor that night.

Uta began to muse about why the ghost was male. In one daydream, the ghost became sad, sat on a branch, and cried. At that moment, Uta became aware that the ghost had turned into a female. The transference aspect of this transformation is extremely interesting, as the analyst's name, Ast, means "branch" in German. Earlier, by seating the then-male ghost on the "branch," Uta was accomplishing interrelated psychological processes, symbolically joining father (male ghost) and mother (female ghost/branch/Ast) images to create a different pair of parents and thereby maintaining her generational position as the child instead of being stimulated to take the mother's place with the father. Now, the ghost who turned into a sad woman represented a part of Uta (she called it her "soul"), who could now sit on Dr. Ast's lap (on the branch) and be nurtured in a way different than her biological and depressed mother had nurtured her. After this daydream, Uta did not mention the ghost in her sessions other than to refer to it as a sad woman.

One night soon thereafter Uta awoke from her sleep and found that she had been crying. She sensed that her "soul" had been crying. She was having a more appropriate (sad) response to her childhood traumas and the surrender of some childhood identifications and object-images. Much later, Uta would say that her analysis taught her to mourn over the missing maternal love of her developmental years.

A Period of Enactments

While Uta was experiencing these psychic changes, she remained with the sculptor boyfriend. Her interactions with him were, however, still under the influence of her internal processes. Around this time, Uta was selected to be one of the "ladies" at an event reenacting a medieval marriage ceremony to attract tourists and to be shown on television. As was the custom, the "ladies" would ride horses through the streets surrounded by "peasant women." But she could not accept being cast as a "lady" and instead chose to participate in the ceremony as a peasant woman. Several hours later, she had unprotected intercourse with a bisexual man who, she knew, was at risk for AIDS. Uta's fantasy was to become a carrier of AIDS so that she could infect her sculptor boyfriend, who, like Bryan, came from a well-to-do Aryan family; her thoughts were not on her own possible death but on revenge. By killing the sculptor, she would rob an "Aryan" family of their "most precious possession": their beloved child. This constellation of events coalesced her desire to avenge the atrocities perpetrated by the Aryan overclass on her nomadic, "peasant" people.

In the fourth year of her analysis, Uta was able to reveal the details of her sex life with the sculptor, which eerily echoed the circumstances of her developmental years. She told Dr. Ast that they never kissed and never had intercourse face-to-face; he would approach her from behind in the way that she had fantasized her father having sex with the family dog. Furthermore, Uta and the sculptor slept in two different beds in the same room, as she and her father had done when she was a girl. And the two habitually masturbated simultaneously in their separate beds, much as she had masturbated in her bed as a girl while fantasizing that her father was masturbating. Uta began to understand that her relationships with different men were connected to her childhood developmental issues and that her sex life reenacted internalized object relations that were pathological. Learning that she used sex with various men for other purposes, particularly that she had reenacted her oedipal child bedroom scene with her latest boyfriend, she separated from the sculptor, but not before their interactions recalled the violence in the "Gypsy" side of her childhood family and imagined perils of her dangerous oedipal father. The sculptor, who had not been violent with her before, struck her in the face, breaking her glasses, and tried to choke her in the midst of a heated argument. Uta came to her next session with Dr. Ast with bruises on her face. After this session Uta never saw the sculptor again.

Freed, to some extent, from expending her energies in enactments of her internalized object relations and psychosexual conflicts, Uta turned them substantially toward the transference with Dr. Ast, expressing a desire to trust Dr. Ast even more. Uta was a Traveler/Gypsy, however, and Dr. Ast was a German and thus belonged to the group that had persecuted and victimized her people; Uta was, as yet, unable to discuss this aspect of their relationship with genuine affect. As she was separating from the sculptor, she began to "kill" Dr. Ast, too, 5 minutes at a time, by regularly coming 5 minutes late to her sessions. She reported that she was late because she had squandered her time drinking tea before getting on the subway to her analyst's office. Dr. Ast eventually interpreted Uta's tardiness to her as a reflection of her angry, depressed mother's tea-drinking, and the enactment ceased.

Shortly after Uta resumed her full sessions, however, she began to have anxiety attacks while traveling. Of course, the concept of "traveling" was rife with meaning, as Jenish people are often called "Travelers," so Dr. Ast suggested to Uta that her anxiety might be yet another reflection of her people's historical legacy. In response to this revelation about her anxiety attacks, Uta became actively interested in knowing what had happened to her parents during the Nazi period. Uta, who had moved into her own apartment shortly after starting analysis, began to visit her parents' house and there to repeat aspects of her childhood experiences, even as she sought to learn more about her parents' past. For instance, she slept in one room but left open the door to an adjacent room where her mother slept, as had been the arrangement when Uta was a child. As they lay in bed, the two women talked to each other before falling asleep; Uta asked about her mother's childhood, especially her life under the Third Reich, but the answers she received were vague. As Uta listened, she developed the fantasy that her mother had been raped by a Nazi or a German.

The frustration of her search for direct answers about her parents' lives during the Third Reich also culminated in a peculiar behavior pattern, another type of enactment. Unbeknownst to Dr. Ast, Uta had once more begun to sleep with many different men. As Dr. Ast was soon to discover, Uta had chosen her new boyfriends according to their first names. All of the men had first names starting with "Ma," such as Mark, Marcus, Marius, or Martin. During her analytic session, Uta referred to these men as "Ma." Knowing that Uta always called her mother "Ma," Dr. Ast quickly deduced the dominant meaning of Uta's new group of boyfriends: They represented her mother's image, to which she related with ambivalence; she wanted to repair them, but she also wanted to hurt them. Since the men were "Germans" in reality, she, like her mother, wanted to become an extension of their Aryanness, but their "black spots" (bad behavior) also kept them in place as "Gypsies."

Uta's method of choosing her companions according to certain criteria, such as their first names, also seemed to be modeled on the Nazis' selection of categories of people for extermination. This idea brought to the analysis a parallel observation. In order to become an analyzand, Uta had stopped being a "nomad"—had changed her city and left the job that required constant traveling. Uta's new job also required that she "select" individuals to perform certain tasks based on certain categories—according to their ethnic backgrounds and physical appearances. It now occurred to Dr. Ast that perhaps Uta, out of fear of being discovered to be a Gypsy (victim) by her German (persecutor) analyst, had split off and projected her Gypsiness onto these individuals and had thus secretly become identified with the Nazis. When Uta eventually understood this meaning of her job change, her investment in her new job was effectively sublimated. Uta decided that because she was well-paid, she would continue in her job—which, indeed, had opened up many new opportunities for her.

As the meanings of her new multiple sexual affairs emerged, Uta once more began to speak of her "Aryan–Gypsy" conflict. Dr. Ast had long been aware of Uta's lifelong propensity to handle her conflicts through enactment, so it came as no surprise when Uta reverted to actions to "recall" an influence of the Third Reich in her internal world. Uta's new enactment also involved finding a new "Aryan" partner whose name started with "Ma." But this man was different from Uta's other choices because he behaved like a *Herrenmensch* (member of the "master race"), treating others as if they were *Untermenschen* (lower human beings destined to serve the master race). Apparently possessed of a narcissistic personality organization infused with certain malignant elements, he made racist remarks about people of color and ostentatiously exhibited his muscular body. Uta saw him, as she understood later, as a symbolic representative of a true "master race," as a neo-Nazi. She often wished to have sex with him all day until the two of them "merged." She also wished to become pregnant by him and to mother his baby. Until recently (about 4 years into her analysis), she had maintained an unrealistic conviction that she could never become pregnant, so developing the idea that she could have a baby did have some progressive aspects. When her relationship with the neo-Nazi was examined in analysis, however, a deeper significance to her extra-analytic transference reaction to this man surfaced.

The Nazis had considered Gypsies' and Travelers' genetic structure to be inferior. Such individuals—via the principle of *Erbkranker Nachwuchs* (Hitler, 1930; Kuhn, Staemmler, and Burgdorfer, 1938), the passing of genetically initiated illnesses to one's offspring—would only produce offspring who would be prone to mental deficiency, antisocial activities, alcoholism, and other undesirable "Gypsy qualities." If such people were allowed to propagate and proliferate, in the Nazi view, they would become a threat to the Aryan populations, who possessed high-quality character traits. Uta consciously believed that if she had a baby, she would pass only "bad things" to her child and actually seemed to think that because she was a carrier of "bad traits," she could not get pregnant. Interestingly, Uta was not at this time aware of the Nazi ideas and policies pertaining to sterilization, promoted as early as 1933, which in fact had their origin in the notion of *Erbkranker Nachwuchs*. Accordingly, Dr. Ast suggested to Uta that through her wish to get pregnant by her neo-Nazi boyfriend, she might be trying to reverse a historical event: trying to compel the Nazis to make nomadic women pregnant rather than sterilizing them. Dr. Ast also interpreted Uta's wish to merge with an Aryan/(neo-)Nazi as standing also for her wish to fuse the analyst and the analyzand; becoming pregnant would be a trial identification with her analyst/mother. During such a process, neither the German nor the Jenish would be killed, or both would be killed, depending on perspective.

After this session, Uta was afraid that she might be pregnant. If she were, she wanted to obtain an abortion, though this desire would also signify that another Gypsy's baby could be killed—another form of sterilization/extermination that would identify Uta with the Nazi victimizer. She was also hesitant to maintain her identification with Dr. Ast. Uta was not pregnant, however, and soon stopped seeing the neo-Nazi. The night that she took the pregnancy test, she had the following dream: "I am bleeding through my vagina, and I am lying in a pool of blood between my legs." Indeed, eyewitness accounts of forced sterilizations powerfully echo Uta's dream; Zdenka Nedvedova-Nejedla, who was interned in Auschwitz, describes, "I tended the children the whole night after the operation. All these girls were bleeding from between their legs and in such pain that I had to secretly give them painkillers" (Fings, Heuss, and Sparing,

1997, p. 94). Soon after reporting this dream, Uta unrepressed a number of remarkable childhood memories. When she was a child, her mother had taken her to visit a neighbor who had been sterilized by the Nazis, not a Gypsy, but a woman with a slight mental disability. Now Uta remembered that she had imagined the sterilization process and had been shocked and afraid. During her adolescence, terrifying thoughts about sterilization had remained in her awareness, but were later repressed. Uta could not recall whether her mother had given her details of how nomadic women were sterilized by their tormentors, but she later learned that her mother's village of origin was quite close to one of the Nazis' sterilization centers.

Uta now also recalled that when she was about 11, she had read in school that Jews and Gypsies had been persecuted, sterilized, and murdered during the Nazi era. At the time, she recalled, she had consciously wished not to be associated with the persecuted groups. This experience probably contributed to her adolescent refusal to visit her father's family—who, as we mentioned previously, lived in a trailer park as "Gypsies." Two years after reading about the sterilization of Jews and Gypsies, Uta "accidentally" cut her labia with a razor while shaving her pubic area. After this event, she was conscious for many years of believing that her genitals were deformed. The meaning of a story that Uta had told earlier in her analysis now appeared in a new light. When Uta was one and a half years old, her upper lip had been cut when she accidentally fell from a baby carriage. She did not actually recall this incident; her parents had told Uta this story when she was growing up, emphasizing that barbed wire had cut her upper lip—but, she remembered, making no association to "barbed wire." Now, Uta could connect the mental images of her two cutting incidents: These images "verified" her nomadic identity and the Nazi persecution of her people. Understanding this fact permitted her to give up symptoms that she had had as an adult: experiencing vaginal pain during sexual intercourse and acute cramps in her lower abdomen whenever she saw on television a person suddenly being cut or mutilated. As she became conscious of a link between her vaginal and lower abdominal pain and her image of women sterilized during the Third Reich, her symptoms disappeared.

A Review Dream

After Uta came to understand that she had been enacting her traumatic developmental experiences and defenses against them and that she often perceived such experiences through a lens of conflicts pertaining to her large-group identity and the legacy of the Third Reich, Uta's transference relationship with Dr. Ast intensified. Uta, now at the beginning of the fifth year of her analysis, decided that nothing more was to be gained on the couch; she demanded that her analysis be terminated. Dr. Ast sensed that their therapeutic alliance now allowed

Uta to experience her analyst as "a true Nazi" in her transference neurosis; as Uta became more invested in being a "Traveler," she wanted to escape from Dr. Ast.

Uta decided to terminate on the November day when, in Germany, the dead are remembered and honored, a day on which it is customary for people to place flowers on the graves of relatives and friends. Associating enabled her to understand certain meanings of her choice of date. First, she wanted to bury the images of her depressed mother and her mother's sister. Second, and most important, she wanted to bury her aggression, which was also associated with the Nazis. Third, Uta's wish to terminate on a day when the dead were honored was also related to her internalized image of Bryan; because he was buried in a private walled cemetery, Uta could not visit his grave. She believed that if she finished her analysis on the memorial day, she would be free of the images of the dead and her aggression and could "begin life" all over again. Dr. Ast understood that the way Uta wanted to finish her analysis would still be a form of enactment; it would be magical. She suggested that if Uta did not attempt a magical death followed by a fantasized rebirth—that is, if she remained in analysis—she might have an experience in which a German and a Jenish could genuinely relate to one another without the anticipated conflicts and anxieties. Uta, Dr. Ast suggested, might benefit from the experiential knowledge that a settled German and a Jenish could be in the same room three times a week without persecution.

Uta elected to stay in analysis and began to reveal to Dr. Ast more freely her investments in nomadic identity. She was excited to learn more about Gypsies and Travelers and to share this newly discovered knowledge with Dr. Ast. Eager to know more about her still-"speechless" parents' experiences under the Third Reich, she visited an uncle, one of her father's brothers, who acquainted her with their Jenish ancestors and their one specifically Gypsy branch. Her uncle also told her that her father had never forgotten his first wife and recounted past times when he, Uta's father, and his first wife had gone together to social gatherings where they sang, laughed, smoked, and drank. It is interesting that although Uta's uncle gave her information about the family, he, too, was "silent" about his and other Travelers' and Gypsies' experiences under the Third Reich. But this uncle made it clear to Uta that if someone called him *Zigeuner* in a disparaging fashion, he would take umbrage and defend himself. Presently, he had a good German boss who was protective of him, and he in turn worked hard for his boss; the uncle owned a house and several apartments and considered himself wealthy. In this uncle, Uta had found a "good" father figure with whom she could laugh and talk about their ancestors in a nonderogatory way. This nonconflictual bond with her uncle would slowly be transferred to Uta's biological father, allowing her to get to know and enjoy him. After a great deal of work in her analysis, Uta's relationship with this uncle also helped her to accept certain elements of her self-images as a Traveler and a Gypsy with more comfort.

For instance, with her increased comfort with her Traveler images, her wish for rhinoplastic surgery had completely disappeared.

Around this time, Uta brought to one of her sessions what might be considered a "review dream" (Glover, 1955). In Uta's dream, Bryan appeared carrying a piece of paper with a list of items on it, including the words *wedding gown*: he and Uta were going to be married. Together they went to a house, which looked like a combination of Uta's present apartment and her parents' house. Through the open windows, a storm wind blew into the house, which was filled with white linen. The linens that had covered the furniture flew about in a whirlwind. Eventually, the linens fell to the floor in disorder. After the storm passed, Bryan left the house, leaving Uta behind with two men in the background. Uta saw Bryan going over a tunnel-like wooden covered bridge, and she knew that he was returning to his own house, that he was not going to marry her.

Uta and Dr. Ast spoke of how Uta no longer needed to cover her background under white linen. Her analytic work had created a whirlwind in her mind, leading to the development of a modified internal structure. She was also clearly separating a "Gypsy" house from the house Bryan was returning to (an "Aryan" house). But her separation of nomadic people from settled Germans was different now from the one she had used when she began her analysis. Initially, her identity as a Traveler was conflictual, and she wanted to deny and repress it while attempting to associate herself with "Aryanness." Now Uta, feeling more comfortable with her large-group identity, was separating it from "ordinary" German identity in order to cherish it. When, in the dream, Bryan left, she remained with the two men whom she identified as her father and her brother—Jenish-speaking people whom she was now more and more accepting as part of herself. Uta now spoke without embarrassment or anxiety of how her father and brother at times stole minor items; even her mother would take things of little value that did not belong to her if she thought no one was looking. The covered bridge represented Bryan's casket, but further association revealed that the safe-looking bridge, because it was made of wood (Ast/branch), also stood for the analytic process that had helped Uta to separate herself from wished-for and defensively held Aryanness—from Bryan. Furthermore, she mentioned, her brother, who suffered from infrequent epileptic attacks, had learned to trust a German neurologist as Uta had learned to trust Dr. Ast.

As a child, a normal oedipal passage had been denied to her. Now, Uta began to develop a new relationship with her father and to enjoy his company immensely. Furthermore, she gave up having multiple sex partners and began to speak about finding a suitable man for a lasting relationship. As Uta resolved to finish her analysis without urgency, she began speaking about three men whom she knew and comparing their character traits. One of the men was the neo-Nazi by whom Uta had wanted to have a baby (the "bad" German). The second person was an older ethnic German man, for whom her mother had worked as a cleaning woman. He was a sophisticated gentleman who sometimes visited Uta and conversed with her on various topics, but who never used Uta for sex (the "good" German). The third man was someone with whom Uta could relax and laugh (the nomadic person). The analyst suggested that the different character traits of these men represented aspects of Uta that she was trying to integrate by seeking a partner who combined the characteristics of these three men.

Uta responded to this suggestion in a dream, which she brought to her next session. In the dream, she was in a classroom talking with a teacher who represented Dr. Ast. Uta and the teacher were examining the topic of "air." But at Uta's initiation, they began to study the subject of "marble." One cannot touch air, Uta associated; it is untouchable just as Gypsies were considered "untouchable." She also associated air with gas—the gas used to exterminate Jews and Gypsies and other undesirables at the camps. "Marble," on the other hand, was something solid that could be refined and crafted into a work of art. Uta sensed that her identity was solidifying, a process she attributed to the increased trust that she had established with Dr. Ast and the developing ability to integrate various aspects of herself.

Watching President Bill Clinton's impeachment trial in the U.S. Senate on German television provided the day's residue for another dream. In this dream, Uta was in the White House, a place that she had never visited in reality. Surrounded by other people, she sensed that she occupied a high position in the White House, but not the presidency. Her associations to this dream reflected her hidden power to destroy a man through sex, as well as her attempts to integrate her sense of self. In German the words *White House* (*Weißes Haus*) and *orphanage* (*Waisenhaus*) sound similar; indeed, as Uta began reporting her dream, Dr. Ast thought that Uta was speaking of being in an orphanage. With her increased ability to interpret her internal world, Uta quickly joined Dr. Ast in understanding that she was attempting to put together her "Aryan" and "Gypsy" sides. The White House stood for Aryanness, idealized Germanness. She could accept being in the White House, but she could not allow herself to be the top person there, just as she could not tolerate being a "lady" in the medieval marriage ceremony, but instead had opted to remain a "peasant woman." Like Monica Lewinsky, she could hurt the top person; she could be a Gypsy taking revenge on the powerful oedipal father/white establishment. Uta could talk freely now, without anxiety, about her attempts at integration.

Comparing Uta to an immigrant, Dr. Ast used the psychoanalytic understanding of the psychology of immigrants—whether they move to a new country of their own volition or are forced to emigrate (Grinberg and Grinberg, 1989; Volkan, 1979, 1993)—to illustrate to Uta what she had done to resolve her identity conflicts and to solidify her new sense of identity. When immigrants adapt to a new country in a nonconflictual manner, their new identity is neither a total surrender to the new culture nor the sum of the two cultures. The new identity reflects those selective identifications with the new culture that can be harmoniously integrated or proven congruent with the cultural heritage of the past; the immigrant experiences what Salman Akhtar (1995, 1999) calls a "third individuation." Uta was confident that she could now choose what to keep from Jenishness, as well as from Germanness, and what to discard of those aspects that were defensively established and infused with the legacy of the Third Reich.

The Deaths of Uta's Father and Uncle

As Dr. Ast and Uta began to discuss the possibility of terminating her analysis, now in its fifth year, Uta had a peculiar experience. During a visit to her parental home, as usual, her father put his arms around her. Since she had become close to her father, Uta had responded to her father with affection, but with no sexual feelings. This time, however, she found herself experiencing conscious sexual arousal. After reporting this event to Dr. Ast, Uta began to realize that her experience was a sign of her progress in analysis. Her prominent unconscious fantasy that included the Third Reich images, if it could be translated into words, might read as follows: "Because I am a Gypsy, I am sterilized and I cannot have a child. Therefore, I can act out my oedipal fantasies in a much safer way and experience sexual feelings for my oedipal father, whose nightly presence in my bedroom stimulated me. Because I am sterile, I can also handle my competition with my mother well." Uta had reacted to this unconscious fantasy in two ways: First, as a child, she repressed and denied having sexual feelings for her father; second, as an adult, she became promiscuous, having sex with men who became mere numbers. Experiencing open sexual desire for her father, however transiently, then, was an indication that Uta was giving up her repression and denial and facing a previously anxiety-inducing wish. After this incident, in fact, Uta and her father formed an even stronger father–daughter relationship, for which her earlier closeness to her uncle had prepared her. Uta's affection for her father also created a new comfort in her relationship with her mother. For the first time in 25 years, Uta took a picture of her parents together. Symbolically, she was putting her parents together and enjoying them. She had solidified as a postoedipal child who had given up oedipal strivings.

Most unfortunately, at the peak of enjoying her life without anxiety and guilt, Uta experienced a terrible loss: Her father suddenly died. Even though his health had been failing for over a year, the death was unexpected. A week after her father's death, Uta's uncle, who had cancer, also died. The loss of these two men reactivated Uta's grief over Bryan's death and the impending separation from Dr. Ast. But she had no fantasy that she had caused her father's death or her uncle's and was grateful that she had felt close to them before they died.

At this time, a seemingly insignificant event occurred that provided Uta with a profound insight into her own large-group identity and into ethnic relations in general. A few weeks after the deaths of her father and uncle, Uta, though not a devoutly religious person, decided to visit the church she had attended with her parents when she was a child. While in the church, she found herself crying openly. A woman who appeared to be from the Far East approached Uta, proffering a written prayer and praying beads. The woman explained that if Uta read the prayer and used the beads, she would feel better. Although Uta was touched and genuinely appreciative of this woman's attempt to assuage her grief, she decided not to follow the advice—though so as not to be insensitive to the woman's kind gesture, Uta accepted the items. The thought occurred to her, however, that people from two "different worlds"—people with vastly different cultural and religious heritages—could have safe, warm human interactions. At the same time, she began to feel better about living in Germany as a Traveler. Free of the influence of Third Reich images in her representational world, she could now blend these heretofore antithetical images—German and Jenish—into an identity that was enriched by both.

Termination Phase

After her acute grief over losing her father and uncle subsided, Uta truly began the termination phase of her analysis toward the end of its fifth year; as is typical, she revisited conflictual issues of the past for one last review and working-through. Uta recontacted her former neo-Nazi boyfriend and began to have sex with him. Through this affair, she was revisiting her earlier "Gypsy-German" conflict. Since Uta already understood this conflict, Dr. Ast remained silent, allowing Uta to work through this aspect of her "symptom" on her own. In spite of understanding their renewed relationship as a symptom of her resistance to termination, though, Uta did not stop seeing the neo-Nazi and having sex with him. Instead, she became involved in an unusual pattern of behavior: She had fellatio with this man in a public place very close to where she worked. If they were caught, they would both be humiliated. Uta had never done anything like this before and wondered what she was trying to tell her analyst by her unusual action. On the one hand, she was Monica Lewinsky, taking revenge on a powerful Aryan, but, on the other, she was showing Dr. Ast that she was a stereotypical Gypsy, a truly "low-class" person, by having sex in a public place. She spoke at length about this renewed relationship in her sessions, "waving" the details of it before Dr. Ast as though they were a red flag. Uta was trying to demonstrate that she still needed the analyst's help, asking Dr. Ast not to leave her.

Uta came to realize that on the surface, she was re-differentiating, at the termination phase, her large-group identity from the large-group identity of the analyst: a revisitation of the separation-individuation issues. Slowly, though, more poignant meanings emerged. Uta, as a Traveler, wanted to express her love and gratitude to a German, Dr. Ast, before they said "goodbye" to each other. She had found this a most difficult task; she could not openly mourn the loss of a

German with whom she had developed a loving attachment. Uta's stereotypical Gypsy behavior was a way of denying her tender feelings about Dr. Ast. On the other hand, she was also forcing Dr. Ast to decide whether or not she would still accept and care for a "real Gypsy" who had done something that would be unacceptable for a "real German." Since the "real German"/Nazi boyfriend was also involved in this activity, though, she not only made herself a stereotypical Gypsy, but also, in a sense, tried to show her German analyst that there was no difference between them. If she were still "loved" by Dr. Ast, Uta could at last believe, once and for all, in a "good" relationship between Gypsies and Germans. With this realization, Uta allowed herself to mourn the coming termination of her work with Dr. Ast and discarded the neo-Nazi boyfriend.

After losing her husband, Uta's mother could not grieve properly; she was trapped in anger. During a visit to her mother's home, Uta found herself its target. The temperature was very high that day, and Uta's mother felt hot, both physically and emotionally. Instead of responding to her in a negative manner, Uta fetched a pail of cool water for her mother. Uta's mother calmed down upon soaking her feet in the water and responded positively to her daughter's gesture. She asked Uta to join her, and Uta took off her shoes. As the two women sat side by side, soaking their feet and cooling themselves, Uta helped her mother talk about memories of and feelings for Uta's father. In a sense, Uta was able to put her mother's mourning process on the right track by identifying with Dr. Ast, who had helped her to learn how to mourn. Uta's mother had rarely uttered kind words to her daughter, but now expressed her happiness over Uta's visit and asked Uta to come again. On the train back to her apartment, Uta reported, she had experienced a kind of reverie. First she compared Dr. Ast with her mother; then she imagined that she had given her hand to her analyst, who held her hand in return. This image, she knew, symbolized her analysis. By holding Dr. Ast's hand, Uta was able to revisit her whole life and to prepare for a more comfortable future; she felt satisfied with her analytic work. Upon hearing this, Dr. Ast also felt satisfied—and noted her own sadness about letting Uta go.

During the rest of their work together, Uta recalled many "memories" of her analysis in a "work of mourning" (Freud, 1917b) for her relationship with Dr. Ast, who would soon become a "lost object." Among her reviews, she looked back at her use of Third Reich and related ethnic symbols to express her internal conflicts. Now she knew that she had, without being fully aware of it, spoken Rotwelsch as her initial resistance to analysis, creating a kind of linguistic haze between herself and her analyst. Instead of hiding the differences between the analyst's large-group identity and her own, she now wanted to compare identities in a playful fashion.

Uta asked Dr. Ast where the analyst's "soul" was located. Dr. Ast thought that she and perhaps most Germans would point to their heads. Uta responded that she and other Jenish women would typically think of their souls as located in their vaginas. Through sterilization, then, the Nazis had crushed Travelers' souls. Uta now realized that, in turn, in another history-related unconscious fantasy linked to her other unconscious fantasy of Gypsy sterilization, she had used her vagina as a kind of annihilation camp to take revenge on the Nazis. She would "select" 50 or so Aryan men, as the Nazis chose individuals for sterilization or the gas chambers. She would have sex with them once or a few times without love or genuine attachment, turn them into "numbers," dehumanize them, and discard them. Now, Uta wanted to use her soul, her vagina, for libidinal purposes. She described her vagina as a place where life could be passed on from one generation to the next and declared her newfound sense of womanhood very dear to her. From now on, she would choose partners based on these new values.

Reviewing the meaning of "selecting" people by ethnic and other criteria, Uta once more changed her job. She received a promotion in the company where she worked; her job no longer involved selecting people from various ethnic backgrounds for various tasks. Outside of her sessions, she enjoyed her life and success at work, and she also deepened her relationships with women friends, a new experience for Uta.

Before completing her analysis, Uta repainted, with her mother's permission, parts of her parents' house in vibrant colors. Her father had done such jobs when he was alive; by carrying on with his tasks, she felt close to his image and, at the same time, came to enjoy her mother's company. The two women began to take walks together in the woods, something that they had never done before. Uta now was a postoedipal person, and Dr. Ast herself felt like a proud mother, pleased to see Uta happy and blooming.

Uta's case will be discussed further in chapter 11, which deals with therapeutic techniques for individuals who bear Third Reich images. Now the remarkable story will be told of a German psychoanalyst, "Sabine," who also carried parental images related to traumas suffered during the Nazi period.

8

Sabine

A GERMAN WOMAN'S "SELF-ANALYSIS"

Born in 1950s West Germany to a mother who had been adopted as a child and a father who was a World War II veteran, Sabine is now a practicing psychoanalyst living in Germany. Only after her private practice had begun to flourish did she notice that something was missing in her therapeutic activities: Neither the ethnic German nor the non-German patients on her couch spoke about their parents' activities during the Nazi regime. As she considered this fact, she realized that a corresponding discontinuity had occurred in her own training analysis—in spite of the fact that she and her analyst, who is Jewish, had discussed her father's presumed Nazi membership on a number of occasions. In order to illuminate this dark territory, Sabine began a postanalytic journey of "self-analysis." This chapter details that remarkable journey, illustrating the degree to which the mental representation of the Third Reich could settle in Sabine's mind even though her father and mother had remained almost entirely silent about their experiences.

Sabine's Mother and Father

Thirteen years of age when the war ended, Sabine's mother, Brigitte, had, as a child, participated in the Bund Deutscher Mädchen (literally, "German League of Girls") organization, the girls' equivalent of the Hitler Youth. Indeed, she had enjoyed it. Such "clubs" (really, official organizations) provided a sense of belonging to children, helping them to loosen ties to their families and to identify with a group of peers. The young people went on excursions, sang songs, and participated in exercises not only to enhance their group sense of belonging, but also, in accord with Nazi ideology, to exclude outsiders as "antisocials." As National Socialists and Aryans, the children were taught, they were supposed to give up their own individual needs for the benefit of the community. Because Sabine's mother was an adopted child, taking part in the Nazi youth group might well have given her a sense of belonging that was missing in her family life.

Later, during her adolescence, Brigitte blamed her adoptive mother (Sabine's grandmother) for not teaching her to be critical of the Nazi regime. Indeed, Brigitte did not learn about the atrocities of the concentration camps until the end of the war, even though her adoptive father was serving as a major in the Wehrmacht (the German Army) in the East. Strangely enough, however, as Brigitte was told after the war, her family had given sanctuary to a Jewish man during the war. Although she had not directly understood at the time that her family was harboring a fugitive, Brigitte later recalled having vaguely felt that some sort of secret existed in their apartment sometime during the war years. After the war, Brigitte learned about the mass murder from some American soldiers who showed her photographs of prisoners in the death camps. Realizing that by participating in the Nazi youth organization, she had been ideologically prepared to belong to the group that had committed those crimes, she was terrified by the sight of those pictures, as she later told Sabine.

The family of Sabine's father, Klaus, who was 23 years old at the end of the war, had originally lived in Czechoslovakia, where they owned a farm. Klaus's father, the oldest son of his family, had been captured during World War I and was forced to work in a mill as a prisoner of war in Russia. After the war, the daughter of the mill's owner had wanted to marry Klaus's father, but he instead returned to the family home in Czechoslovakia. Traditionally, the oldest son was to take over the family farm; because no one had heard from Klaus's father for many years, his younger brother had managed the property in his absence. The younger son, however, did not now turn the farm over to Klaus's father, as might have been expected; we do not know whether any sort of struggle occurred between them on this issue. But Klaus's father soon left the farm for a nearby city. While Klaus's father was in training to become a professional butcher, his younger brother committed suicide. Family members believed that the brother had killed himself because he felt conflicted about not giving up stewardship of the farm to his older brother. In turn, we speculate, Klaus's father might have felt that he had "killed" his own brother by returning home. He nevertheless returned to the farm, got married, had three children, and became a butcher. Klaus was the oldest child, born in 1922; he had a brother five years younger and a sister who was the youngest child of the family. Although, among professionals, horse butchering was regarded as the nadir of the profession, Klaus's father became quite wealthy by selling cheap horsemeat during the postwar period, when most people were too poor to buy beef.

When the Austro-Hungarian Empire collapsed after World War I, Czechoslovakia, which included old German settlements, emerged as a separate state. A large number of Germans, including Klaus's family, remained in their settlements. As Klaus was growing up, ethnic Czechs began to pressure German-speaking people in Czechoslovakia to assimilate more fully. Germans were "encouraged" to change their German names to Czech ones; ethnic Czechs were favored for loans; and people with German surnames were refused jobs in state-run organizations. Unsurprisingly, German nationalism among those ethnic Germans living in Czechoslovakia simultaneously increased, and Klaus's family was no exception—its members were proud of their German heritage. As Czech and German nationalisms made the two groups into enemies, Klaus's father sent his oldest son to live with a Czech family on the principle that learning the Czech language would be good for the family business. Klaus's association with a Czech family, however, did not prevent him from developing nationalist attitudes. He was a member, and eventually a leader, of the local German Youth Sports Association—which, after the German occupation and annexation of part of Czechoslovakia, became the Hitler Youth.

When Klaus entered the army in 1939, his brother was only 13 years old. Just before the war ended, the brother, now 17, quickly trained as an SS soldier and was sent to the Russian front. His job was to jump into enemy foxholes and, as the family myth phrases it, to "butcher" the Soviet soldiers with a bayonet. After the war, he recounted vivid memories of his time in Russia to his elder brother. He reported knowing that if he refused to perform his task, the SS officers would shoot him on the spot. In 1948, while training to become a butcher himself, he cut an artery with a knife while skinning an animal. Even though a hospital was just across the street from the place where he worked, his life could not be saved. The family myth also suggests that the younger brother could not live with his memories of "butchering" the fur-capped Russians, and that his fatal accident was in fact not an accident, but a suicide. The history of the previous generation appears to have repeated itself: a younger brother commits suicide, while the older one survives.

Before enlisting in the German Army, Klaus had attended an engineering high school and had planned to study engineering further. During the war, he worked in a factory, helping to develop machine-guns for fighter planes and working on the mechanics of dropping bombs from airplanes. He occasionally flew in warplanes himself as an engineer, mostly on missions in the Soviet Union. During its productive years, the factory to which Klaus was assigned included among its personnel workers who by night were detained in a heavily guarded camp nearby. Sabine now believes that they were probably slave laborers brought from concentration camps. When she spoke with him about these workers several years ago, however, Klaus insisted that they "must have been criminals because they were imprisoned." It appears that even in 1998, Klaus continued to believe in the Nazi "justice system" on some level.

Sabine's Story

Klaus survived the war and married Brigitte in 1952, four years after his brother's presumed suicide. They eventually had three daughters, of whom Sabine is the youngest; one of her sisters is one year older, the other two years older. According to the family story, Brigitte became pregnant for the third time because Klaus wanted to have a son, and Klaus did not go to the hospital to see his newborn daughter for several days after her birth. We conjecture that Klaus wished that Sabine had not been born—that she were either dead or male. Paradoxically, however, it is clear that, in Klaus's mind, Sabine was a special child. Probably out of guilt for his initial response, Klaus made Sabine a special being from an early age. Later, however, other events also rendered Sabine the special one among the three children.

According to Sabine's mother, after this "disappointment" to her husband and his family their marriage began to fall apart. In truth, however, Brigitte and Klaus's union had been shaky from the beginning. Just before they married, Sabine's parents decided to buy a puppy. The day of their wedding, the puppy, soiled and without water, arrived in a small cage. Brigitte somehow believed that her husband was responsible for caging the animal and perceived him as "cruel" toward helpless, weak beings, as she continued to think for years to come. During her formal analysis, Sabine came to the conclusion that as an adopted child, her mother identified with the caged puppy. Acting like a kind of "adopted bride," she related to her husband as if he represented her adoptive parents; she did not belong to her environment, and the caretakers (her parents, her husband) were cruel. Later in their marriage, Brigitte continually complained to the children that their father did not provide enough money for them to be fed or clothed properly; again, the caretaker was a callous agent of deprivation.

When Sabine was 6 years old, her parents separated, though they remained married. Klaus left Germany to work in Africa, whence he was to send money to his family. Eventually, Klaus returned to Germany and found employment in a city distant from the one where his wife and children lived. Sabine's parents finally divorced when she was 13. Later, her mother married a foreign national and left Germany. Her father remained in Germany and married another German woman. Neither parent had other children.

As a little girl, Sabine was very active; indeed, she was quite an intrepid child, taking risks while swimming or skiing without apparent anxiety. Another of her early passions was riding; from the age of 5, Sabine loved horses. A year after Klaus returned from Africa, however, she was kicked in the head by a horse. For a few days, it was uncertain whether 11-year-old Sabine would survive this accident. Of course, she did live, but experiences mild difficulty breathing through her nose to this day. Though otherwise she bears no scars on her face from the accident, she vividly recalls studying her smashed face in the car mirror on the way to the hospital as if fascinated with what she saw.

Although Sabine excelled in school as a teenager, during her adolescence she became aware of a disturbing symptom: She frequently felt that she was destined to die at any moment. Although she never planned suicide, a sense of the nearness of death remained in her mind constantly. Later, Sabine studied medicine simply to "fill up time," as she thought of it, before her imminent demise. Later she realized that she had felt like a prisoner condemned to death. Learning medicine was an attempt to find an escape from her fate; she would cure her patients, who, by displacement, stood in for her. In her medical studies, she was extremely attentive to minute details because, as she reasoned, such precision might make the difference between life and death for a patient (or herself). At the same time, Sabine felt that her own fate was irrevocable. Her sense of inevitable destiny and her constant striving to escape that destiny went hand in hand.

After becoming a physician, Sabine began her psychoanalytic instruction, including the conventional training analysis with a senior analyst, through which Sabine was better able to understand a number of the significant events of her youth. For instance, Sabine was taken to a child psychotherapist at a very young age to investigate why she continued to speak in "baby talk" past the age of 4. (Indeed, her earliest memory is of "shooting" at this psychotherapist with a toy gun.) Though Sabine does not remember the event herself, Brigitte has told her that one day she simply stopped talking like a baby and began to speak clearly in perfect full sentences. During her training analysis, Sabine connected her "baby talk" to the fact that her mother had been adopted at the age of 18 months. In fact, it was a complete mystery to Brigitte how she had spent the first year of her life. It is possible that Sabine's mother had transmitted images of her own troubled childhood to her daughter and that the young Sabine felt she had to remain baby-like in order to resolve on her mother's behalf what Brigitte had deposited into her. The analyst also related Sabine's constant feeling of impending death to Brigitte's early abandonment. He interpreted Sabine's dread as an expression partly of her mother's sense of peril and partly of Sabine's own anxiety about losing her mother. Discovering this connection was a great relief for Sabine.

It should be noted that, during her formal analysis, Sabine and her analyst did not explore Klaus's possible role in the development of these symptoms. But they did spend a great deal of time investigating his role in the incident with the horse. First, Sabine realized that for some unconscious reason, she had caused the accident. Usually, trainers use a long whip that they crack from a distance to prompt the animal to behave in certain ways; the accident had occurred because Sabine had no whip that day. Though, by the age of 11, she was already an expert at handling horses, on that day she hit the horse's back with her hand without warning it. Startled, the horse kicked Sabine in the face.

Sabine came to recognize that the accident was related to her disruptive identification with her mother, who herself had been kicked by a horse when she was 12 years old, breaking her nose. Furthermore, Sabine realized, her own role in the accident was connected with guilt feelings surrounding her oedipal issues; she had, in a sense, replaced her absent father with her horse. Facilitating this replacement was Sabine's parents' fondness for horses, which might have included reaction formation on Klaus's part. As a child, he had been ashamed of his family business—which, it will be remembered, was butchering horses; as an adult, he encouraged his daughters to ride horses, as the children of upper-class families would do. Her parents' increasing marital difficulties further stimulated Sabine's oedipal wishes. Early in her "adolescent passage" (Blos, 1979), in the midst of the process of unconsciously re-examining her oedipal strivings, she joined her sisters and her embittered, disaffected mother in constructing a monstrous image of her father. She split the loved image of him away and affixed it to the horse, loving it as an oedipal daughter loves her father. Finally, she ended up punishing herself for her oedipal wishes by causing the accident, provoking the horse (the father-representative) to reject her; her displaced libidinal object, instead of loving her, almost killed her.

Thus it became clear to Sabine that preoedipal and oedipal fantasies contributed to her significant experiences and symptoms. As her analytic work progressed, Sabine experienced an affective discharge about her sense of fatality, and the conviction that she would die soon suddenly disappeared before Sabine could gain an intellectual understanding of her symptom's multiple meanings. She and her analyst decided to terminate her analysis, agreeing that they had worked together successfully as much as they could. Soon after terminating her analysis, however, Sabine began to have the feeling that something more needed to be resolved.

Sabine's analyst is a German Jew who managed to survive the Holocaust by hiding for several years within Germany. His wife, who was also persecuted during the Third Reich era, was one of Sabine's favorite professors in medical school. Sabine eventually understood her involvement with the couple as related to her own conflicted oedipal issues, her search for "good" parents, and her perceptions of the analyst as a "good" father and of his wife as a nurturing mother. During her analysis, however, images of the Nazi era began to appear in dreams and fantasies connected with her transference neurosis. In one dream, she imagined her analyst was being sent to Auschwitz. When she felt guilty for this expression of murderous impulses toward her analyst, she pictured, in another dream, young women washing themselves in a bathroom; in the dream, she knew that they were in a death camp and that the young women would be gassed in this bathroom. Identifying with the women, Sabine defensively made herself a victim.

Looking back, Sabine feels that her anxiety about identifying with the Nazis was something that she and her analyst could speak about but not fully explore and work through. Furthermore, Sabine and her analyst examined Sabine's image of her father as a Nazi, but not as a traumatized person himself. They did not examine the possibility that she had served as a reservoir for his traumatized self-images connected to hidden war experiences. Furthermore, she felt she could not speak freely about transference anger toward her analyst since the anger of a German toward a Jew seemed, by definition, murderous. Repressing her anger, she experienced him for an extended period during their work as "a nothing"—in her words, "like air." Looking back, Sabine realizes that this notion might be related to both her wish to annihilate (to gas) her analyst, as well as her wish to give him a means of survival (air to breathe). Through her long silences, she tried to make him a nonentity, to annihilate him, psychologically speaking. But the analyst tolerated and "survived" Sabine's silence-attacks.

A year after ending analysis, she felt an urge to see her analyst and made an appointment to see him. When he asked why she had returned, she told him that they had not fully discussed the fact that he was a Jew and she the daughter of a Nazi. Sabine's analyst seemed astonished, reminding her that they had indeed spoken about such matters "several times." But he also acknowledged that his Jewish identity and Sabine's German identity had made analysis more difficult. After this visit with her analyst, Sabine felt determined to find other ways to understand the legacy of Nazism within herself.

From her teen years until her analysis, Sabine was often flooded with images associated with the Holocaust. Whenever she saw freight trains, for example, she would be reminded of the deportation of the Jews. She was aware of no other person who felt the same way, perhaps because people in Germany, in general, did not (and still do not) speak to others about such private imaginings. Not knowing why she possessed such images, Sabine began to fantasize that her father had done "bad" things during the war, and she sometimes imagined prosecuting him in court. Sabine felt ashamed of having a Nazi father and assumed that he had been involved in atrocities during the war—even though, at this point, she had no factual information about his war activities. Indeed, throughout her childhood and most of her adulthood, Sabine knew little of what her father had done during the war, for Klaus was silent on these matters. But Sabine nevertheless persistently thought of him as a "bad Nazi," for, as she absorbed her mother and sisters' bad opinion of Klaus as a husband and father, Sabine projected onto him the image of the cruel Nazi created by her mother's oft-repeated account of seeing Holocaust victim photographs for the first time. Of course, Klaus's ongoing silence on the subject of his war experiences helped to feed the grim impressions that Sabine formed about him. Once, to her surprise, Sabine's 10-year-old nephew repeated a nationalistic rhyme that he said he had heard from Klaus: "*Schwarz, rot, gelb: deutscher Held. Blau, weiss, blau: tschechische Sau*" ("Black, red, yellow [the colors of the German flag]: German hero. Blue, white, blue [the colors of the Czech flag]: Czech pig"). Sabine was furious, but, when confronted, Klaus simply said that this rhyme had been a common saying when he himself was his grandson's age.

Gonda Scheffel-Baars (1998) notes that some children of Nazis and collaborators, out of unconscious resistances to their parents, remain in a stage of rebellion and develop their own life "programs" that are contrary to their parents' behavior and belief systems. Sabine's adult behavior reflected a number of such "contra-programs." She was involved for eight years with a Jewish man from Israel, to whom she remained loyal even when his family refused to accept her because she was German. Eventually, he, too, rejected her and married a Jewish woman. She refused to take part in group activities where an enthusiastic crowd would gather, struggling to dis-identify with the Nazi murderers—while, in her fantasy, her father was one of "them" all the time. On occasion, she consciously felt that as a German, she herself might do bad things if she were not careful. As a defense against the shame and anxiety of associating herself with the aggressor, as well as against oedipal closeness with her father, she believes, Sabine was able to develop only the most fleeting conscious feelings of nationalistic pride. More routinely, she disassociated herself from Germans during national events—cheering, for example, for any team competing against West Germany in the Olympics.

Until she embarked on her "self-analysis," she remained apparently distant from her father; whenever Klaus attempted to be generous toward Sabine—by providing additional financial assistance, for example—she refused his support. Still, she was conscious of her identification with him in certain areas; her speech patterns were nearly identical to his, for instance, and, like him, she usually waited until the last minute to catch a train. As she was to learn over the coming years, the true extent of her identification with him was far more profound.

The Reunification of Germany: A Catalyst

As the German Democratic Republic ("East Germany") and the Federal Republic of Germany ("West Germany") prepared to reunify in 1990, Sabine became increasingly concerned that rampant anti-Semitism would reappear as an outgrowth of renewed German nationalism. Sabine sensed, even at the time, that the reunification of Germany generated such anxiety for her because the threat of revivifying the Nazi monster symbolized the return of the "bad" East German/oedipal father who had abandoned his daughter by going to Africa. Since Sabine was in the termination phase of her formal analysis during the period of reunification, she could not explore fully with her analyst what the historic event meant to her. Nevertheless, reunification did prompt her to ask Klaus about World War II in an effort to get to know her "real" father, despite her anxiety about what she might discover. He responded simply that he had been an engineer who enjoyed technical challenges, an intellectualized response that did not offer Sabine much information about the specific nature of his activities during the Nazi period or his feelings about them. Finally, she asked him to join her in watching *Shoah*, the acclaimed documentary about the Holocaust. After watching the film with Sabine, he finally began to talk. "Yes," he said, "I was in a camp like that." Sabine was terrified that he would say he had been a guard at such a camp. Instead, Klaus remarked that he had been a *prisoner* in a camp like the one in the film. It was the first time that Sabine had realized that the war might have been quite difficult and painful for him. She wanted to feel sorry for him, but she found that she could not yet allow herself to feel empathy for a former Nazi soldier.

A year after the reunification of Germany and the end of her formal analysis, she met Dr. Volkan and Dr. Ast—who, at the time, were investigating the ways in which mental images of the 1989 collapse of the Berlin Wall and the subsequent reunification of Germany echoed in the self-concepts of individuals affected by those events. Through psychoanalytic interviews, including exploration of subjects' developmental issues, adaptations to mental conflicts, and symptom formation, Dr. Volkan and Dr. Ast were evaluating reflections of these events in their subjects' fantasies and dreams (Ast, 1991). Sabine volunteered to take part in the study and soon became interested in Dr. Volkan's research on the transgenerational transmission of trauma. Wondering if there were reasons for her horse accident other than oedipal guilt, and not yet realizing that her father might have played a role in the other symptoms outlined earlier in this chapter, she embarked on a "self-analysis."

She knew that when Freud's (1887–1902) letters to Wilhelm Fliess were discovered and examined carefully, the concept of "self-analysis" had assumed a new meaning, for now Freud could be seen to have examined his own internal, unconscious world through a transference relationship with Fliess. No longer did "self-analysis" designate an isolated investigation of one's own dreams and thoughts alone. As Freud (1925) wrote in his *Autobiographical Study*,

> It must not be supposed . . . that transference is created by analysis and does not occur apart from it. Transference is merely uncovered and isolated by analysis. It is a universal phenomenon of the human mind . . . and in fact dominates the whole of each person's relations to his human environment. (p. 42)

No serious self-analysis can take place without finding someone to whom to address it. For Sabine, that "someone" was Dr. Volkan; without noticing it at first, Sabine evolved a transference relationship with Dr. Volkan. Perhaps his Turkish ethnicity was a factor in this development; in her private practice, Sabine had treated some Turks living in Germany and was aware that they were now the "new Jews" in her country. Perhaps, too, the fact that Dr. Volkan was neither German nor Jewish helped Sabine to perceive him as a "new object"—as separate from her early developmental conflicts. In any case, Dr. Volkan told Sabine he suspected that her Jewish analyst had credited her perception of a horrible and criminal Nazi father because of the analyst's own experiences as a German Jew during the Third Reich era. Sabine realized that her self-analysis would benefit immensely if Klaus ended his own silence. The task of helping him to overcome that reticence was forbidding in itself, however, because it required her to modify her own long-held, monodimensional image of her father. Her formal analysis—which was most useful in other ways, and which had explored and resolved many of her object-relations conflicts, early identifications, and oedipal issues—had not necessarily prepared her to develop a more realistic view of Klaus. Frequently in contact with Dr. Volkan, Sabine would spend over six years in the process of developing a new understanding of her father—and a new understanding of herself.

While driving with Sabine in the countryside one day, Klaus began to speak about his and his brother's involvement in the war; now Sabine learned new details of the stories we reported earlier in this chapter. For instance, Klaus had taken part in evacuating wounded German soldiers from Soviet Army–surrounded Stalingrad in 1942. Klaus vividly remembered some men clinging onto an airplane over-weighted with other casualties. As the plane took off, the men let go and fell to the ground, and Klaus recalled pushing some wounded German soldiers from the airplane so that it could take off. Sabine immediately felt that these images had haunted Klaus throughout the years.

As Klaus continued to speak, Sabine realized that his world had collapsed when he was captured by the Soviets in 1945. When the Allies' triumph began in earnest, the regular German soldiers who protected the factory where Klaus worked were replaced by about a thousand old men and adolescents—a rather motley "regiment" that Klaus was ordered to lead. But almost all of the old men and children were killed in Soviet attacks, and Klaus himself was taken prisoner and confined to a single cell. Now he recalled to Sabine feeling shocked to realize that he did not understand the world anymore. He had been an engineer and was prepared neither to command the defense of the factory nor to see people die. Being German, being a National Socialist, being obedient to authority, being a soldier/engineer—these had all been highly valued qualifications. Suddenly, he was imprisoned and waiting to die for possessing those same qualifications. Indeed, prison life itself had violated his sense of the world. He was given food in a metal pot and told to defecate in the same pot after he ate; after emptying his feces, his captors put his next meal in the same dirty pot. Each day, Klaus was told that more prisoners had been killed and that his time would come soon; for three weeks, Klaus awaited execution. But his mind was constantly occupied with finding an escape from his hopeless situation. Finally, it occurred to him that since he spoke perfect Czech, he could convince his captors that he was Czech and not German. The ruse worked; he was released.

Instead of seeking safe refuge, though, he took many risks to return to the family farm in Czechoslovakia, just as his father had done after World War I. Klaus set to work in the family business as if there had been no war. Looking back, Klaus now realized that his own father was aware of the foolishness—even the danger—of resettling his eldest son on the family farm. The war was over, but everyone who still lived in the area knew that Klaus had been a leader in the

Hitler Youth. About six months after his return, Czech civil guards appeared on the family farm—among them, people from their own village, his father's customers—asking for Klaus. He hid in a closet, but to no avail; he was taken, with other Germans, to a train station. The group of Germans was herded onto a freight train with no idea of their destination: a former Nazi concentration camp. Now the tables were turned: The prisoners were German, and the guards were Czechs.

As a former leader of the Hitler Youth, Klaus received a form of "special treatment": The Czechs imprisoned him in a hole in the ground covered with some sort of door; in effect, he was buried alive. In imagining the psychological effects of this bizarre form of torture, we are reminded of Otto Fenichel's (1945) remarks on "foxhole waiting":

> The blocking of external motor activity increases the probability of a breakdown, and foxhole waiting [in Klaus's case, waiting in a dark pit with an expected death sentence] is more dangerous than active warfare. (p. 117)

Each morning, before the other prisoners awoke, Klaus was taken out of his hole for a "special task": He was to collect and bury the corpses of German prisoners who had been killed during the night by drunken Czech guards. Some Germans' skulls were smashed from beatings, and Klaus was forced to clean up their brains. Knowing this history, Sabine was less shocked that Klaus would remember—and pass on to his grandson—a bigoted rhyme about Czechs.

Many months after he was captured, on a day when Klaus was not confined to what Sabine calls his "burial place," he was selected by a Soviet officer to work outside of the camp because he still looked young and strong enough for hard physical labor. Somehow, he managed to escape from the work detail. From there, Klaus fled to Austria, where he was once more captured by the Soviets and jailed for a third time. Eventually, he regained his freedom, and, at the age of 30, married Sabine's mother in Germany. Only three years later, Sabine was born.

After listening to her father's war stories, Sabine began to realize that her expectation of impending death had held other significance. Originally, as it turned out, it had been not Sabine, but Klaus, who "knew" that his death was approaching. Now she saw that she had been the reservoir for a paternal self-image traumatized by the *actual* experience of awaiting imminent death. Sabine recalled that when her symptom first arose during adolescence, she would have the sensation of "falling into a hole," feeling hopeless and panicky. At the same time, Sabine realized that Klaus—by externalizing his traumatized self-image into his daughter's developing self-image—had freed himself from his burden. Accordingly, he had been able to build a reasonably happy and fruitful life with his second wife. Furthermore, Sabine began to think that her accident—in which the horse had kicked her in the head—might be connected to her father's experience of collecting and burying corpses with smashed heads.

Klaus's story of Czech torture also recalled for Sabine a dream that he had reportedly had soon after Sabine's birth, a dream about which Brigitte had told Sabine when she was an adolescent. In the dream, he saw holes in the ground from which rabbits were trying to come out, and he was trying to push the rabbits back into their holes. Even at the time, Brigitte said, she herself understood her husband's dream as the expression of a wish that Sabine had not been born—a wish that Sabine should die, as psychoanalysts would recognize it. In each of the two previous generations before Sabine's birth, a younger brother had killed himself; it seemed as if one out of the three children in each generation was destined to die. In Sabine's generation, it appears that the death of the third-born daughter was also expected. Indeed, upon hearing of his daughter's equine accident, Klaus anticipated that she would die and brought a black suit for her funeral with him from the city where he worked.

At this point, Sabine recalled her sister having discovered Klaus's old letters from Africa in her basement several years previously, while Sabine was still in training to become a psychoanalyst. Klaus himself later recalled addressing all his letters from Africa to Sabine, the special child, and, in fact, although he had written to other members of the family as well, many of the letters were indeed sent to the prepubescent Sabine. What is most intriguing about these letters is that in almost all of those addressed to Sabine, Klaus writes constantly about death-related themes, death rituals, and events in which someone dies. On one occasion, he even relates to 8-year-old Sabine a true story in which a father leaves his 8-year-old daughter for a short trip and never returns because of a fatal accident. In this almost obsessive thematic repetition, he seems to have unwittingly been preparing her for imminent death—his or hers.

Why, however, besides being the unwanted daughter, was she chosen by her father to be a reservoir for unwanted self-images linked to his traumatic experiences? Sabine found a possible answer to this question when Klaus told her of an event that took place during the first week of her life. When he finally allowed himself to go to the hospital to visit his newborn daughter, he discovered her not breathing, turning blue. He thought that Sabine was definitely going to die, but he held her by her feet upside down and shook her—as they had done with baby animals on the family farm back in Czechoslovakia—to help her breathe again. Klaus, in essence, brought her back to life. Having verged upon death, Sabine had apparently become an appropriate repository for her father's externalization of his own image as someone waiting to die in the prison camp. It is likely, furthermore, that Klaus's externalizations played a role in another of her childhood symptoms: her prolonged babyhood. If little Sabine were going to die in any event, in his mind, she did not need to speak in fully formed words and sentences or to grow up; she needed to stay victim-like for Klaus. We may further speculate that Klaus, hearkening back to his Nazi days, might also have perceived his "victim" daughter as being like a Czech or a Jew who "needed" to be victimized or killed—though, of course, we have no way of confirming this last possibility. What we do know is that at the age of 4, as was mentioned earlier in the chapter, Sabine suddenly ceased to baby-talk after directing her aggression against her psychotherapist with a toy gun. After hearing her father's war stories, Sabine began to think of this earliest memory as an expression of killing a prison sentry to gain her freedom, as if the imprisoned father within her needed to shoot his guard in order to reach safety. Feeling safe, little Sabine could then begin to talk, but the imprisoned-father image stayed within her. By depositing his own "waiting to die" image into her, Klaus caused her to feel that her own death was imminent.

As she pondered this psychological reality, Sabine began to understand why Klaus sometimes insisted on giving her certain items. For instance, when she bought a house, her father insisted on giving her a toilet that was in his house so that he could buy a new one. Sabine had no need for this old toilet, and at first she found Klaus's request unusual, if not bizarre. After talking with him, however, she sensed the urgency of his effort to discard the old toilet. It was as if Klaus wanted to deposit his old "bad" feelings, memories, and victim-images (symbolized by the toilet/feces) into Sabine's self-representation (symbolized by her house). Sabine acceded to Klaus's request in order not to hurt his feelings, but she never installed the toilet. Another item Klaus wanted to give his daughter was an old sailing boat that he had kept for 25 years but had never used. Sabine was convinced that this boat, although beautiful, was unsafe: The boom was too long and seemed to her to be placed lower than it should be. Sabine politely refused to take it, but her father insisted. As she reflected on her fear that the boom would smash her in the head or knock her into the water, she at once vividly imagined the smashed heads of Germans from her father's village. Finally, she took the boat as a gift, but never ventured to sail it. Whenever Sabine tried not to accept a gift from her father, the expression on his face would change as if he were going to have a temper tantrum, which Sabine now interpreted as his response to her refusal to be a reservoir for his intolerable discarded (externalized) self- and object-images. But on both of the occasions mentioned here, she nevertheless accepted the gifts, though she did not use them.

As Sabine gradually discerned the unconscious interactions between them during her developmental years and throughout her life, she began to try to free herself from serving as a reservoir for her father's unwanted self- and object-images. For a time, she even entertained the idea of explaining to him that he had unconsciously used her as a reservoir for his traumatized images of himself as a prisoner of war and the associated object-images he had internalized. Perhaps she could show him that he had needed to externalize the image of corpses with smashed heads, for instance, in order to give himself internal relief from aggression against his captors, as well as from his helplessness, humiliation, and guilt. But Sabine gave up the idea of telling Klaus about what he had done unconsciously because she thought that at the age of 76, he might not be willing or able to understand. Furthermore, she knew that by employing his daughter as a reservoir, he had made himself "free" to enjoy life. More important, she decided, was for her to work through the influence of what had been deposited in her without returning the images to her father.

What was missing in Sabine's understanding at this point was the idea that Klaus might associate his own traumatized self-images with images of the Nazis' victims, a possibility that Dr. Volkan suggested to her in a later conversation. If Klaus did make such associations, he never spoke about it, nor did he ever openly express any remorse about what the Nazis had done to their victims. Her father's previously unspoken sorrow seemed to be connected only to his own suffering and the suffering of his fellow countrymen—and, perhaps, to the lost "grandiosity" of Nazi Germany.

A "Second Look" at Czechoslovakia

As Sabine differentiated herself from what her father had deposited into her self-representation, she found herself enjoying Klaus's company more and more, and he responded enthusiastically to their changing relationship. As she came to appreciate how much her father had suffered after the war, her rebellion and counter-identification gave way to empathy and, to some extent, forgiveness; he had, she concluded, been "punished" enough. Gradually, she even began to accept and to appreciate his financial assistance. At the end of the sixth year of Sabine's "self-analysis," she and her father spontaneously embarked on what, in the clinical literature, is known as a "second look" activity.

The concept of *second look* was first formulated by Samuel Novey in 1968. Novey wondered why some patients in psychoanalysis have an urge to explore old diaries and papers and to return to the physical settings and persons important to them in an earlier phase of their lives. His first conclusion was that these activities should be differentiated from "acting out"—performing a repressed memory, mental representation, or affect rather than verbalizing it in analytic hours. An example of "acting out": A patient reacted to his analyst's vacation by taking a vacation himself, a holiday that he spent sitting in a hotel room looking at a particular breast-shaped mountain. Analysis of his behavior later revealed that his analyst's vacation had induced in him "memories" of oral dependency, his mental representation of a nurturing mother, and the affect of longing for such a mother-representation. Instead of allowing himself to be conscious of his oral dependency and longing for his mother/analyst's breast, the patient claimed to have no reaction to his analyst's absence. After analysis of his behavior, however, the patient allowed himself to experience genuine feelings about his oral dependency and its transference manifestation.

By contrast, prior to a second-look activity, individuals first recall the previously repressed material and acknowledge the importance of that material in their psychic make-up. They then enact the second look in the service of working through the previously repressed conflicts. Though a second look is an action, rather than a therapeutic verbalization, "it constitutes behaviors in the interest of furthering the collection of affectively charged data and thus helping the treatment process" (Novey, 1968, p. 87). Similarly, some travels made, against inner resistance, in order to master internal conflicts can constitute a kind of second look, even if unconnected with an ongoing analysis. If the pilgrim already possesses a strong observing ego that can use action in the service of its integrative functions, such a journey can be successful; Warren Poland (1977) and Ira Brenner (1999a) describe several such pilgrimages in detail. Indeed, a successful pilgrimage to a personally significant site can sometimes resolve transgenerational conflict (Volkan, 1979) by leading to the mastery of conflicts unconsciously harbored by the parent, which, in turn, have become part of the traveler's unconscious heritage. This, indeed, is what Sabine and her father were able to achieve.

Sabine asked her father to accompany her on a trip to the Czech Republic to see the place where their ancestors had lived. Klaus agreed, and the two of them drove from Germany to the village where Sabine's grandparents' farm had been. The trip took many hours, during which the father shared more "memories" of his childhood and of the Third Reich. When they arrived in the village, Sabine observed that a river divides the village into two sections. In the past, she learned, one section was populated by ethnic Germans such as her ancestors, and ethnic Czechs occupied the other section. Now, the situation was different: Both sides of the river were populated by Czechs. Though some individuals in this village still considered themselves Germans, most of them were married to Czechs and were apparently assimilated into the community.

As Klaus and Sabine crossed the bridge that connected the two sections, Klaus recalled that he had returned to this location after the Soviets freed him the first time. He remembered that as he crossed the bridge, he had seen his father on the other side and had immediately noticed the older man's anxiety. The father's first words to his son after so many years were, "How dare you come back!" Klaus told Sabine that he had known that it was "crazy," as he said, to go home, but had felt compelled to return. As they stopped for a time at one spot on the bridge, Klaus began to cry. Sabine was filled with empathy and relief; Klaus was assuming responsibility for his own personal history, and she no longer felt herself to be a reservoir for the image of a father who had expected to die. From the village, they went on to the city where Klaus had been tortured and surveyed the fields from which he had collected the corpses of people he knew. They actually saw a hole in the field, and Klaus wondered whether it was the place where he had been buried alive. Sabine found that she could now externalize the images of dead corpses and her father "buried alive" onto their original location, the place where they had actually existed.

As Klaus and Sabine returned to the village, a man of Klaus's age approached him and said: "I am the Jew—do you remember me?" Klaus did indeed remember this man. In fact, there had been a time, before Klaus's involvement in the Hitler Youth, that they had played together as children. Now, the two men sat together and began to talk. The Jewish man spoke of his parents' deportation and of his own time in Auschwitz. He had returned to Czechoslovakia after the war, and, after retiring many years later, he had returned to their native village, becoming part of the German community there. As the two men recalled their youth in the village and laughed together, Sabine was fascinated to witness Klaus and this Jewish man effecting a kind of reconciliation. Indeed, the man invited Klaus and Sabine to come to the local German church, where he helped the priest with the logistics of serving a large parish. As she observed their reunion, Sabine noticed something else as well. Both Klaus and this Jewish man seemed to experience certain yearnings for the old days. They spoke of the public Christian ceremonies of past times; it seemed, surprisingly, that both men had enjoyed them. They further commiserated, strangely enough, that modern police forces are no longer sufficiently determined to keep the peace by force. The psychodynamics of this situation were certainly far more complex than we can fully understand from the information we have: It is possible that a meeting with a Jewish person from his past had revived for Klaus the feelings he associated with submitting himself to an authoritarian regime; the Jewish man, on the other hand, might certainly have been expressing a form of identification with the aggressor. Regardless, what first startled—and then pleased—Sabine most was the visible reconciliation between the two men, their ability to speak about both "good" and "horrible" events.

Finally, Klaus and Sabine reached their ancestral house, now owned by a Czech family. This family, after learning who the visitors were, invited Sabine and Klaus into their home. As they walked from room to room, Klaus, with great emotion, showed Sabine where he had slept, where her grandparents had worked, and so on. The Czech family invited Sabine and Klaus to join them for beer, and the Germans accepted their offer. And thus a sort of peace was made between Klaus and the Czech people as well. When Sabine and Klaus's pilgrimage to their ancestral village came to an end, they drove back to Germany through the small Czech city of Pribor—the birthplace of Sigmund Freud, the city formerly known as Freiberg—at Sabine's suggestion. Sabine and Klaus visited the house where Freud's mother had given birth to the future "father of psychoanalysis." While drinking coffee near Freud's birthplace, Sabine and her father discussed Freud's life, including the fact that he was Jewish. In the course of their conversation, Sabine described the structure of the unconscious mind and explained how symptoms develop. Klaus, translating her explanation into the language of an engineer, spoke of his understanding of the mind's "construction." The father and daughter had found yet another new link in their relationship. For Sabine, visiting Pribor meant receiving a kind of acceptance or blessing from her "spiritual father," Freud—a sort of sign that her self-analysis had ended.

Klaus, who is quite proud of his psychoanalyst daughter, wanted to please her by accompanying her on a "pilgrimage" to Freud's birthplace, but Sabine sensed that there was another meaning to this side trip as well. For Klaus, it also seemed to be a gesture of appreciation to Sabine's "spiritual father" for playing a role in his daughter's recent closeness to him and his roots, for he acknowledged that Sabine's altered attitude toward him was based in her psychoanalytic experience.

The End of "Self-Analysis"

In a conversation not long after their "pilgrimage" to these two important native places, Klaus wondered aloud why none of his children had wanted to know about his past until Sabine inquired about it. Until then, Sabine had not discussed with Klaus the role that she believed he had played in the development of her symptoms. Now, in an empathic fashion, she tried to explain to her father how the horrors he had seen during the war might have unconsciously been passed on to her. Though she handled her father with sensitivity and respect, part of her very much wanted him to know that she had joined him in his experience of the Nazi regime and of World War II, even though he had not been able to talk about either topic until quite recently. But Sabine quickly saw that it was difficult for her father to have such a conversation. Her father clearly still seemed fixed on his many residual blind spots about the Third Reich, so she changed the subject of conversation. She did not wish to force him, at his age, to confront the profoundly painful images and affects against which he had defended himself for at least half a century.

Soon after this conversation, Brigitte, Klaus and his wife, and other relatives and friends gathered at Sabine's house to celebrate her birthday. Soon, Sabine realized that her father had, in fact, heard or sensed something of what she had been trying to tell him about their unconscious relationship. He spoke about her two near brushes with death and indicated how happy he was that she had survived and had built her own life; he wished her to be happy for the rest of her life. Her father's birthday gift was not bizarre, as some of his gifts had been in the past, but most appropriate; Klaus had prepared an album of photos he had taken during their trip together to the Czech Republic, and on the cover he had written this title: "A Journey to My Natural and Spiritual Fathers' Homeland." Sabine felt an internal peace. At last, she felt, her self-analysis had come to an end; she was content to leave her father with his blind spots.

9

The Psychotherapeutic Study Group for People Affected by the Holocaust

TOWARD ENDING THE "SILENCE" IN GERMANY

IT MAY AT FIRST SEEM STRANGE to speak of Germany's "silence" concerning the Nazi past. After all, hundreds of publications and artistic works have anatomized the period of the Third Reich. The German government has repeatedly acknowledged the crimes of the Nazis in the form of financial compensation, as well as in formal apologies to the Jewish people. In 1970, Chancellor Willy Brandt knelt in contrition, to acclaim at home and abroad, at the Warsaw memorial to Polish victims of the Holocaust. Since the late 1980s, German civic and artistic debate has focused on the question of how best to commemorate the victims of the Holocaust in a gigantic public monument at the heart of Berlin. How, one may ask, can the Germans be said to be silent on the topic of the Third Reich?

When we speak of the German "silence" about the Nazi era, we are referring to a different sort of silence—one that has intimately interpersonal and transgenerationally intrapsychic ramifications. Rather than public debate, we are interested in individuals' use of psychological mechanisms—ranging from intellectualization and rationalization to splitting and denial—that protect self-esteem by establishing emotional distance from aspects of the Third Reich that induce shame and guilt. The collective effect of these individual "silences" tends to keep intellectual understanding segregated from affective responses to the Holocaust as a trauma. Though, over the decades, several investigations have provoked emotionally heated exchange among Germans about the psychological repercussions of the Nazi period, the emotional consequences of those investigations have tended, in the long run, to be denied, dissociated, or isolated.

For example, only a small minority of scholars in Germany has accepted the analysis proposed by Alexander Mitscherlich and Margarete Mitscherlich in 1975 (Moser, 1992; Schneider, 1993). In their well-known work, Mitscherlich and Mitscherlich suggested that Germans avoided psychological association with Hitler and the Nazis by mobilizing enormous shared defenses against guilt, shame, and anxiety. In turn, they argued, these shared defenses prevented the German people from mourning the loss of the Third Reich, especially the loss of the Führer. All one permitted oneself to feel was "an isolated regret for only one's own losses" (p. 41). Because properly mourning the Third Reich would have required the affective survey that would necessarily confront what the regime had done to its victims, the Mitscherlichs concluded, failing to grieve for the loss of the Reich meant that German society never fully appreciated—or mourned—the loss of its victims. German psychoanalyst Burkard Sievers (1999) cites the conservative philosopher Hermann Lübbe (1983) as the most prominent German scholar who has rejected absolutely the idea that German society has been unable to mourn. Lübbe is convinced that former West German Chancellor Konrad Adenauer's (1949–1963) efforts to repress the "memory" of the Nazi past via amnesty and amnesia were essential to consolidating democracy in the Federal Republic of Germany after World War II. Postwar German society had placed a high priority on material, not psychological, rebuilding; working through and coping with the trauma of both victims and victimizers were split off from Germans' conscious efforts to secure the nation's economic footing. For the most part, traumatic war experiences were never really confronted—and, indeed, still wait to be confronted. Sievers joins Timothy Ash (1998) in asserting that the supporters of "forgetting" the Nazi past—precisely what the Mitscherlichs aimed to counteract—are an impressively large majority in Germany.

When the German "silence" is broken suddenly and unexpectedly, the rupture often provokes a strongly negative public reaction. Ira Brenner (1991) relates the story of a high school teacher named Posset from the small Bavarian town of Landsberg who had excavated the ruins of a Nazi-era underground factory with his students, unearthing many Jewish graves (Meyer, 1990). Eventually, Posset and his students discovered that this factory had housed the top-secret Third Reich project code-named *Ringeltaube* ("Ring Dove"). The objective of the *Ringeltaube* scheme was to build the world's first jet, a crucial development for the Nazi war effort. With Himmler's permission, about 30,000 prisoners from Auschwitz and Stütthof were relocated near the Landsberg area in order to work on the secret project. By the end of the war, half of these prisoners had died from starvation, exposure to the elements, and murder; if they were no longer well enough to work, they were sent back to the camps for gassing or cremation. The jet, the Messerschmitt 262, appeared in 1944.

But Posset's relentless efforts to revive the town's wartime history were extremely unpopular among his fellow townspeople, who felt that he was turning Landsberg into "a second Dachau" and scaring away the tourists who came to admire its natural beauty. He and his family were harassed, and Posset was labeled a *Nestbeschmutzer*, someone who "spoils his own nest." As Brenner writes, Posset was thought to be symbolically defecating not only on himself and his fellow townspeople, but also on his whole country: "The national conflict over knowing, remembering, verbalizing, and truly learning from the horrors of World War II is a painful condition which, like an individual with a deep conflict, will not be resolved without treatment" (p. 97). Juxtaposed with the virulent public response in the Posset incident, a debate such as the one surrounding the proposed Holocaust memorial in Berlin, which has itself been heated at times, appears slow and intellectualized.

If the affective "silence" in Germany is thought of as a blanket that covers emotional manifestations of Third Reich–related issues, the wear and tear on this fabric must be noted. Symbolic expressions of Nazi images "pass through" the threadbare places on the "blanket" in a process similar to what psychoanalysts call "the return of the repressed." Unlike intellectual discussions of the Third Reich and the Holocaust—which are carried out in a conscious manner, and in which emotions are controlled through mechanisms of isolation, dissociation, projection, and denial—what passes through the wear and tear of the blanket contains, directly or indirectly, the language and emotions associated with such images.

Breaking through the "silence" of Nazi language with its associated affects provides a striking example of such a symbolic expression, according to German psychoanalyst Dieter Ohlmeier (1990). Under the spell of certain feeling-states—such as extreme sadness or anger—we are cast back to the "primal grounds" of our language, the language that was transmitted to us by our ancestors, Ohlmeier argues. During the Nazi regime, propaganda idealized and promoted the "destructive-narcissistic personality formations" of National Socialist identity via a language that is no longer acceptable in Germany. Under conditions of acute feeling, however, Nazi language may penetrate the strong taboo against its use in such words and phrases as *parasitär* ("parasite"); *Versuchsperson* ("human guinea pig"); *Sonderbehandlung* ("special medical treatment"); *liquidieren* ("liquidate"); *bis zur völligen Vergasung* ("gassed completely"); and *fertigmachen* ("finish off"). For instance, in discussing a weighty business matter, an individual suddenly says, "We must come to a final solution (*Endlösung*) of a this administrative matter," without appearing to notice his words' dark undertones and Nazi associations. Ohlmeier offers another example: After two weeks' stay at the university guest house, Jewish intellectuals from abroad visiting a German university found a note from the German housekeeper, who seemed upset that the guests had left items in their room that were to be discarded. The note said that the guests would be charged 80 Marks for the "filth" left behind. The amount of money would cover the cost of *Sonderreinigung* ("special cleaning"), a term used by the

Nazis to refer to the "purification" of German ethnicity from Jewish, Gypsy, and other unwanted elements.

Nazi language and other symbolic references to the Third Reich have also been observed in dreams, providing further evidence for Erik Erikson's (1954) suggestion that dreams may express a certain ethno-syntonicity. Thus dreams can be windows onto shared images of the Third Reich that one avoids in the conscious state but that nevertheless persist in the unconscious. Ohlmeier, for instance, reports a dream that expresses anxiety through an image of the infamous Nazi medical experiments. A 45-year-old German man who had entered analysis after discovering many "death zones" in himself gave this account of a dream:

> In a brightly lit room, I am lying on an autopsy table. You [the analyst] are standing behind me. You wish to operate on me and use me as an object of experiment, but I cannot stop you. You have a demonic power over me, I am totally in your control. You put a long metal instrument into my mouth, deep into my body, and destroy my internal organs.

The neo-Nazi "skinhead" movement (Rosenthal, 1997; Streeck-Fischer, 1999) itself might also be considered a kind of return of the repressed. Third Reich–related sentiments appear undisguised in the dream of a 17-year-old skinhead (Streeck-Fischer, 1999) who unconsciously equated threats to his own identity with threats against the Nazi regime, the "Thousand-Year Reich." His dream reflected his omnipotent wish to repair internally perceived damage to his self-esteem. In the dream, the young man goes through a "time warp" and ends up in the year 1939. Since he sees himself as an expert of weapons technology, he is received by Hermann Göring at the Nazi Ministry of War, who recognizes the young man's importance. His dream continues:

> With my help, jet planes and hydrogen bombs could be produced in Germany. I became Hermann Göring's right-arm man, and one of the most important leaders of the German Reich. With my help, the German Reich won the war. Poland, France, England, Russia and the United States were defeated and destroyed. One country after another capitulated, danger to the German Reich was averted, the world was led into a "German peace." A German world empire was established with the capital at Germania (formerly Berlin). Because of me, the 1000-year German Empire was founded and the German people won eternal peace. And what became of me? I had a long life to live and took on, after the death of the Führer and Hermann Göring, who became the Führer after Adolf Hitler, the office of the Führer myself. Because of me, the world was saved. (p. 87)

Since the neo-Nazi faction operates in the cultural and political arenas, it forces itself onto public attention. The emotions thereby induced can then be used to "neutralize" the unwanted Nazi sentiments among non-skinhead Germans that the skinhead movement brings into view. For instance, the public might have used the anger it collectively felt toward German skinheads' vicious attacks on "guest workers" (especially, but not solely, Turkish in origin) during the 1990s to support its shared wish to disassociate from the Nazi past. "It is 'they,'" the shared fantasy might run, "the skinheads, who do such bad, racist things, not us"—not the images of ancestors deposited within them.

* * *

In the last chapter, we recounted the long "silence" of Sabine's father, Klaus. His silence is not necessarily a representative model, since his main trauma occurred because he was a prisoner of war, not because he was directly a victimizer or a torturer. Nevertheless, we maintain that his reticence over the years was conditioned by his past commitments to Hitler and to Nazi ideology. A volunteer in the Nazi youth movement and later a soldier in Hitler's army, he might once more have associated himself with the Third Reich—now with feelings of shame and guilt—if he had spoken of his personal history to Sabine or other members of his family. As we saw in chapter 8, Klaus's silence had intimately interpersonal and transgenerationally intrapsychic effects on his daughter. After he ended his silence, both father and daughter became increasingly free to speak about the actual history of the Nazi period, to experience affects related to it, and to relate positively to one another.

This chapter describes five individuals' attempts to breach their own silence. Brought together by a shared personal need to examine their own past histories and German–Jewish issues more broadly, all five individuals are psychoanalysts or psychotherapists living in Germany; two of them are Jewish, the rest ethnic Germans. As these five people began to relate to one another closely, they reactivated their own intrapsychic processes around images of the Third Reich, creating a kind of "laboratory" of German-Jewish relations. Of course, we cannot state with certainty that what we observe in this setting can be generalized to all descendants of those traumatized under the Nazi regime. Other work with which we have been involved—such as Volkan and Ast's interviews with Germans concerning the reunification of Germany—and other researchers' findings already mentioned in this chapter, however, suggest that what we learned in this "laboratory" may have a wider application.

The Road to "The End of Speechlessness?"

For some time now, a number of German and German Jewish psychoanalysts and psychotherapists of the postwar generation have noticed that many patients who are approximately their own age (born around 1950) display a common problem. When these patients try to talk about the lives of their parents or other family members during the years of the Third Reich, or about what it was like to grow up in the shadow of the Holocaust, few, if any, can provide accurate and complete details. As the children of this generation were growing up, their families were almost universally uncommunicative about the Nazi period. Nor was the Third Reich discussed in much depth at school, in church, or anywhere else: None of the patients remembered learning adequately about the Nazis or the Holocaust as a child. A child, for example, might come across a photo in the attic of the family home of a young man in uniform and ask a parent about it. The parent might answer that the photo was of a brother who was killed during the war, but no further details would be given: The curious child's many spoken or unspoken questions were met, essentially, with speechlessness. At some level, people behaved as if the Third Reich, the Second World War, and the Holocaust had never existed (see also Bar-On, 1989). It was typically only much later that these patients learned anything about what happened in Germany in the 1940s or about their families' histories during that time; even then, the older generation volunteered little information.

There were, of course, many allusions to the Nazi period in the books these patients had read as children and young people, but these references typically did not correspond to the readers' personal experiences and psychological processes relating to images of the Third Reich. Indeed, if their curiosity led them to seek out the primary texts of the period, it would be difficult for them to access the Nazis' own words. While preparing the present volume, Dr. Ast decided to read Hitler's *Mein Kampf* and some issues of *Der Stürmer* magazine. To her surprise, she found that the central library in Münich owned only three copies of *Mein Kampf*, and that no public library in Münich owned copies of *Der Stürmer*. Readers were not permitted to check out *Mein Kampf* and could look at a copy only under library supervision. When Dr. Ast made further inquiries about the notorious Nazi-era magazine, she learned that in the Bavarian State Library there is one original paper edition and one on microfiche; again, a reader may only look at these items under supervision. As she later learned, individuals are not even allowed to buy a copy of *Mein Kampf* in Germany.

If there were few available publications that could help to address the genuine psychological experiences of descendants of those who had lived under the Third Reich, there were even fewer places that German people could go to discuss personal issues and psychological problems related to the Nazi era. Because contact between ethnic Germans and German Jews can easily be avoided in everyday life, people are rarely required to expose themselves to the emotional influence of the Nazi past.

In reflecting on the emerging pattern among their patients, some of these German psychoanalysts realized that they, too, had encountered the same sort of silence in their childhood. As Annette Streeck-Fischer (1999) writes,

> I myself belong to the post-war generation that neglected to question its parents or who received confusing answers to those questions asked. In our

> memories appear fragments of an earlier time, e.g., a certain mode of speech, that became comprehensible only against the background of the Nazi past, and which because of denial remains unclear in their continuity. Confusions exist with regard to the time dimensions, the meaning of events, what actually did take place, and so on. (p. 90)

Five such therapists living in the Düsseldorf and Köln areas gradually evolved into a small group that met frequently to confer about their patients. They theorized that many of their patients, even though these individuals had not personally experienced Hitler's regime, were nevertheless significantly affected by it. These five colleagues eventually became the core of an organization called Psychotherapeutischer Arbeitskreis für Betroffene des Holocaust, or "PAKH" (Psychotherapeutic Study Group for People Affected by the Holocaust), which we mentioned in chapter 1.

From the first, even as discussion group, PAKH members had trouble communicating with each other. They wanted to address the problem they had recognized, but formulating specific ways to do so proved difficult. Although they sometimes talked about initiating projects, such as a symposium or a clinic for people who suffered psychological problems related to the Holocaust, they more often became bogged down in technical issues, organizational details concerning PAKH, and other distractions. Finally, one of the five core members of PAKH, Liliane Opher-Cohn—who, like Sabine, had been interviewed by Dr. Volkan for the German reunification project—suggested to her colleagues that perhaps Dr. Volkan could provide some insight into their communication problems.

To Mrs. Opher-Cohn, the fact that Dr. Volkan is neither Jewish nor German and was in no way directly affected by the Holocaust were advantages. Born on the island of Cyprus to Turkish parents, he had emigrated to the United States some 40 years earlier. Furthermore, in addition to his clinical work as a psychoanalyst, for more than 20 years Dr. Volkan had studied large-group psychology, mourning, transgenerational transmission of trauma, and traumatized societies and had worked on many projects in which representatives of ethnic or national "enemy groups" were brought together for prolonged series of extensive, unofficial psychopolitical dialogue. Given this background, she argued, Dr. Volkan seemed a most fitting facilitator for their group.

When Dr. Volkan first met the members of the PAKH core group, he was aware that at least some of the members were dubious about seeking help from an outsider who was neither German nor Jewish. But he also had some doubts of his own. On the one hand, he did not want the meetings to turn into "therapeutic" sessions for individual group members, but, on the other, he was uncertain about PAKH's aims and was therefore concerned about his ability to help the group to advance these. In fact, the members of the core group were themselves unsure of the aims of their organization. Among other matters, the members spoke of trying to open a new dialogue within German society about the

Holocaust and its consequences; from this vague sentiment, the idea of holding a symposium eventually emerged. During the 18-month period in which the group evolved the concept of *Das Ende der Sprachlosigkeit?* ("The End of Speechlessness?") and initiated the necessary organizational arrangements for the conference, Dr. Volkan met with the PAKH core group four times: in February 1997, December 1997, March 1998, and August 1998. Each gathering, except the final one held the day before the symposium, lasted for two days.

In his approach to the core group members, Dr. Volkan decided to rely upon his previous experience in conducting small-group dialogues between representatives of opposing large groups such as Arabs and Israelis (Volkan, 1988, 1997b, 1999a). He has learned that when such representatives are given the "task" (Bion, 1961) of discussing the conflicted relationship between their respective large groups, each "side's" large-group identity assumes primary importance, and discussions increasingly reflect large-group issues rather than individual perspectives. The members of each "side" become spokespersons for their respective large groups and tend to feel that they are under personal attack. Individual stories told in this environment generally narrate what "others" did to "us," reflecting aspects of large-group conflicts and large-group identity difficulties. It typically takes time and effort for participants to understand how they have internalized the conflict between their large groups and how it influences their individual identities and behaviors in deep and pervasive ways. Only then can the participants truly begin to communicate, to understand one another in an effective manner and with sympathy.

The relationships between the five members of PAKH were obviously different from those involved in other dialogues Dr. Volkan had helped to facilitate—between parliamentarians, ambassadors, scholars, and other influential individuals from Russia and people of similar backgrounds and professions from Estonia, for example (Neu and Volkan, 1999; Volkan, 1997b). The members of the PAKH core group are psychoanalytically trained colleagues: people with mutual interests, not enemies. Their German and Jewish parents, grandparents, and relatives, however, had lived in a very different reality. Victims or victimizers, they were enemies, and the generations that have followed them—including our colleagues in the mental health profession, as we saw in Sabine's case—carry this legacy, both consciously and unconsciously. Although half a century had passed, the members of the PAKH core group still embodied the unspeakable trauma of war and annihilation and therefore had—albeit in hidden ways—more in common with contemporary adversaries such as Arabs and Israelis or Russians and Estonians than they wanted to believe. And, of course, they were subject to all of the usual dynamics of small groups (Abse, 1974; Bion, 1961; Foulkes and Anthony, 1957).

Accordingly, at their first meeting, Dr. Volkan told the core group of PAKH that he would focus on its members' personal stories only when these stories reflected German–Jewish issues and that he would try to bring to consciousness the hidden psychological significance of these stories whenever possible. He also told group members that he believed that they would be better equipped to study the shadows of the Holocaust in contemporary German–Jewish relationships if they could come to understand their own anxieties, perceptions, wishes, and defenses pertaining to what their ancestors had passed on to them.

This chapter will not report every event that took place in Dr. Volkan's meetings with the core group, but will focus on representative events that clearly illustrate the group's dynamics and evolution. Some background on the PAKH core group members, however, is necessary:

> One was born in Romania to Jewish parents and had moved to Germany at the age of 12, shortly after the end of the war. Her parents had once been sincere supporters of communism and Marxist-Leninist principles in Romania, but in adulthood their daughter had become preoccupied with what it meant to be Jewish.
>
> The other Jewish member of the core group also had been born outside Germany. When he emigrated from Hungary as a teenager, he immediately perceived the silence about the Holocaust that existed in Germany.
>
> One of the Germans knew that his father, a high church official, had opposed the Nazi movement but had nevertheless become indirectly involved once the Nazis came to power. After the war, the father had wanted to become a psychologist but, on the advice of his friend Carl Jung, remained with the church.
>
> Another of the Germans came from a large family in which there was a secret and subtle attitude of anti-Semitism, although few of its members had been involved with the Third Reich. As an adult, this man often wondered what he would have done if he had been an adult during the Nazi period.
>
> The third German's father had been recruited into the Wehrmacht at the age of 17. As an adult, this member had tried to understand the experiences and feelings of his father's youth and was aware of an internal wish to repair what the Nazis had done to his father, as well as to their victims.

The First Gathering—February 1997: A Symbolic Match

A visit by the German national soccer team to Israel during this first meeting focused the participants' concentration on German–Jewish issues. One Jewish member brought to the gathering a newspaper clipping showing a photograph of the German soccer players' visit to Yad Vashem, the Israeli Holocaust memorial in Jerusalem. Because he was a fan of the German team, he also brought a conflict: Would he cheer for the Germans or the Israelis? Consciously, he wanted the German team to win. But looking at the picture he had brought, he asked: "Does he [the soccer player] *really* know about it?"

By "it," he meant the Holocaust. In fact, no member of the core group uttered the word *Holocaust* during the first gathering; all referred to the Holocaust as "it." Even here, there was a taboo that the members of the PAKH group would not break. But this particular "speechlessness" was the seed from which the theme and title of the 1998 symposium eventually grew. If they were unable actually to say the word *Holocaust*, the members were at least able to consider the subject by analyzing the symbolism of the soccer match—though they were not themselves fully aware of the displacement. The Jewish participant who had wondered about the German player's understanding of the Holocaust reported a tension within himself: He was not sure that he really wanted the German team to win. Each participant looked at the newspaper clipping; one of the ethnic German members spoke. Without any doubt, he wanted the German soccer team to be successful, but this desire—peculiarly, he felt—induced some discomfort in him as well. German soccer players, he said, unlike South Americans, whom he perceived as "finesse" players, played a rougher and more physical game, in which they used size and strength to their advantage. His anxiety stemmed from the concern that the German players would be unnecessarily aggressive toward the Israelis. "This," he said, "would make me feel bad and guilty." Another non-Jewish member wished that the soccer game could be played in a "normal" manner and then repeated his desire for "normal" competition between Germans and Israelis.

Discussing the impending German–Israeli soccer match quickly threw into sharp relief members' anxieties about contact between Germans and Jews. "Beating" the Israelis in an aggressive manner would induce guilt feelings among Germans. But if the German soccer players' own guilt feelings concerning the Holocaust caused them to play in an uncharacteristically docile fashion, they might lose a match to an inferior team; that would also be painful. The German group members' wish to see a "normal" soccer match also reflected a wish to have "normal" contact between the German and Jewish members of the core group—something rendered impossible by the legacy left to them by their parents and grandparents. Dr. Volkan sensed that although they themselves had asked him to "force" them to initiate a deeper level of emotional contact with each other, his presence had induced some anxiety, reflected in body gestures of tension throughout the conversation, because it threatened their repressions of German–Jewish issues.

For over a year before the core group's first meeting with Dr. Volkan, the members had met monthly to try to write protocols for their fledgling organization. They felt that this gathering, with Dr. Volkan present, was different, and their discussion eventually involved more than the symbolic discussion of the soccer match. One participant asserted that in the past, "we were afraid to hear each other's personal motives for coming together." Another participant spoke of his wish "to open a window" to the past, in order to learn how to cope with it. He immediately proceeded to tell those present about his family background; his pride in his German ancestors' accomplishments clearly reflected a sense that he had many unfinished tasks concerning his father's involvement with the Nazis.

One non-Jewish participant spoke of an ethnic German friend who had recently visited Israel. The visit had touched the friend deeply, and he had begun to learn Hebrew and to identify with the Jews. The participant did not respect his friend's identification with "the victim"; he thought that it was a defensive response—that through this identification, his friend was trying to escape from guilt feelings connected to his membership in the victimizer group. The member insisted that he himself would not use such a defensive adaptation. He then proceeded to describe a bothersome, unnameable "thing" deep inside him that sometimes expressed itself through migraine headaches. He affirmed a wish to understand this "thing" further, but hypothesized that it was related to an inner struggle of victimizer–victim images. Thus he acknowledged a sort of identification with the "victim," though he pointedly differentiated it from the overt identification of his friend who had visited Israel.

When this participant finished describing how he perceived his family's involvement with the Nazi regime as a bothersome "thing" within him, a Jewish member of the group remarked that he always felt like a victim. His sense of victimhood, he said, was a "personal identity mark": "If I am a victim, no one will do anything bad to me." One German suggested that his own frequent absences from the core group's monthly meetings might be due to a reluctance to hear himself described as an heir of the victimizers. At the same time he did not really wish to miss their monthly gatherings. "I need contacts that will stabilize my identity as a human being," he said.

In short, the first meeting with the members of the PAKH core group focused on considering each member's own identity in the context of German–Jewish interactions. At the end of the meeting, all the participants watched the German–Israeli soccer match on television together—in silence. The game was indeed played in a "normal" way, and Germany won.

The Second Gathering—December 1997: An Enactment

Ten months later, Dr. Volkan held his second 2-day, 12-hour meeting with the members of the core group. Between visits, he kept abreast of their activities through telephone conversations and fax messages: The core group had begun planning a symposium, but much organizational conflict frequently distracted them from their objective.

As soon as the meeting began, one Jewish participant declared that the core group members were moving "too fast" in making arrangements for their symposium on the Holocaust and German–Jewish interaction. "I am afraid of the consequences," he worried. "If we are not successful, PAKH will suffer." "But," he added, "*I am more afraid that we will be successful.*" This, of course, was an extraordinary and highly charged statement, but Dr. Volkan did not immediately focus on it. Rather, he let others speak on their concerns about practical and organizational considerations, ranging from political responses to the symposium to possible disruptions by neo-Nazi groups or outspoken Jewish persons. Finally, Dr. Volkan reminded the group that one of them had voiced a fear that the symposium would succeed. What did his statement signify?

The members began to picture what a "successful" meeting would look like and why it might induce anxiety in one of their own members. A successful meeting, they concluded, would mean genuine emotional contact between ethnic Germans and Jews, especially between the ethnic German and Jewish members of the core group. As Dr. Volkan pointed out, such a rapprochement might entail tremendous risks for both German and Jewish members of the group. Both "sides" had developed certain perceptions about the other, and about the Third Reich and the Holocaust, through the mental images passed to them by their ancestors. Genuine emotional contact with the "other" might threaten the validity of such perceptions and feelings on an individual level and might thus open cracks through which feelings of guilt, shame, grief, rage, helplessness, and entitlement could leak. For each member, the very foundations of individual and large-group identity—the mental representation of both real and fantasized fathers and mothers, and of the fatherland and motherland—could be threatened.

It soon became apparent to Dr. Volkan that the members of the core group had, not long before this second meeting, reenacted quite dramatically what their ancestors had deposited in them about the Nazi regime and the Holocaust, though they were not yet consciously aware that the recent discord constituted such a reenactment. Now, recalling what had happened, they brought—without even being aware of it at first—their transgenerational conflicts to the meeting room so that Dr. Volkan could witness the enactment and interpret its meaning for them.

One of the Jewish members of the group had recently gone to visit his mother and had asked the other Jewish member to accompany him. They told the man's mother that they were going to show their "Jewishness" publicly by participating in an upcoming symposium. She responded by telling the younger people how proud she was of them, but the Jewish woman PAKH member sensed that the older woman, through her nonverbal behavior, was also telling her: "It is better to hide." It is difficult to know, of course, whether the younger woman accurately perceived the older woman's fears or merely projected her own fears onto her colleague's mother. Regardless, the fears of two generations were intertwined (a mini-"time collapse") in the younger woman's response. Meanwhile, the son himself also felt anxious about participating in the symposium, though for apparently different reasons that turned out to be, at a deeper level, quite similar indeed. Consciously, he felt that if he were involved in preparing the symposium, he would not have enough time for his daughter and that the child would suffer. Intensely protective of his daughter, he also feared that involving himself in German-Jewish issues could endanger his family: an echo of the peril Jewish families faced under the Third Reich.

At a PAKH core group organizational meeting not long after this visit, the German members accused the female Jewish member of trying to gain fame and fortune through the symposium. In her perception, their accusation stereotyped her as a "Jewish money-grubber." After the meeting, she called the other Jewish member of the core group—who had been absent—and told him her view of what had happened: Germans were harassing Jews again. He, in turn, became very upset. Unsurprisingly, the Jewish woman PAKH member came to the group's subsequent meeting with much anxiety, unconsciously expecting her present German colleagues to behave like Nazis from the past. In fact, one German participant remembered later that she appeared defensive and tried to dominate the group. A quandary based in the entanglement of past and present thus emerged. The ethnic Germans wished her to behave differently, but they found it difficult to express this desire. Feeling that she was entitled to some sympathy as a representative of the "victim" group, the German members hesitated to assert themselves by opposing her plans directly and openly. If they expressed the aggravation they felt toward her, they would be identifying themselves with the Nazis—which would simultaneously fulfill her expectation that they would behave like Nazis. Finally, one of the German members could not contain his frustration and reacted by stereotyping her. Another German member tried to soothe the tension, using the words *sound and smoke*—the German equivalent to the English phrase "much ado about nothing"—to tell her that her fuss was unnecessary. The Jewish woman immediately associated the phrase, especially the word *smoke*, with Auschwitz and accused him of being a Nazi. At this point, he felt both angry and guilty—angry to be associated with Hitler and guilty because of the association. He wanted to curse at her aloud, but this impulse only amplified his sense of guilt. And so he was struck *speechless*.

With Dr. Volkan present, the members recollected these events as if they had happened moments before and emotionally relived them once again. When everyone calmed down, one ethnic German bravely admitted that when the Jewish woman associated him with the Nazis, he had been stirred to prejudice. Deep down, he confessed, he must still be biased against Jews, even though consciously he wished to be so different. Recalling to the group the wish that its members had expressed to see a "normal" soccer match between the German and the Israeli soccer teams, Dr. Volkan suggested that through preparations for the symposium, another "not-normal" game was being played out between the Jewish and the ethnic German members. It appeared that in the process of trying to establish genuine emotional contact among the members of the core group, they had reactivated malignant but previously hidden German-Jewish interactions. The fear of having a "successful" symposium, he proposed, was the fear of that reactivation. Their contact with each other could induce a time collapse in which mental images of the past—and perceptions, feelings, deeds, and defenses against them—would be condensed with current events, perceptions, feelings, deeds, and defenses pertaining to them. Unpleasant as it might be to contemplate, they should expect shame and guilt, senses of victimization and entitlement, and other conflictual wishes and painful insights to surface, for their large-group identities and chosen traumas shaped their individual behavior. As the meeting progressed, members were able to identify several examples of inherited mental representations of the "other" that had been reactivated during the recent incident. They were beginning to understand how profoundly the past and their present had become intertwined.

During this episode, the female Jewish member had associated her ethnic German friend with a Nazi during the most heated moments of emotional conflict. When her friend insisted on remaining a "good" German by staying calm, she tried to induce aggression, even hatred, in him so that he would "become" a Nazi. On a conscious level, of course, she knew that her friend was not a Nazi; under stressful conditions, however, she unconsciously felt the need to maintain and to reinforce her "inherited" large-group identity as a Jew (and thus as a victim)—and, correspondingly, to sustain the identity of Germans as victimizers. In the meeting with Dr. Volkan, the Jewish woman member did grasp her nondifferentiation of past and present Germans, reporting that after she thought she was being stereotyped as an avaricious Jew, she had felt an impulse to cry out to her mother (who had been dead for 20 years): "Mommy, Mommy! They blame me for killing Jesus."

Ethnic German members also experienced a sense of nondifferentiation between their current identities and their identities as reservoirs of their parents' real or fantasized behavior toward Jews. One of them said of a recent visit to Dachau, "I couldn't stand it." He wanted to run away, to disassociate himself from Germans of the previous generation. But he did not—could not—run away. "I am a German," he continued. "In my name 'it' [the Holocaust] happened. It's no use to run away." He felt ashamed of the impulse toward generational continuity, but also of the impulse away from it as well. Another ethnic German member had visited a Holocaust museum during a trip to the United States between Dr. Volkan's first and second visits. What had affected him most in the museum was a picture of a lost Jewish child searching for her mother. Since this member's own mother had been hospitalized and absent from his life for years when he was a little boy, he easily identified with the little girl's horror of being separated from her mother. His experience of identification at the museum engendered much internal emotional conflict, however, when he returned to a context in which he was associated with the victimizer group.

Differentiating between 1997 and the Nazi period turned out to be a chronic problem for the group, and other psychological processes further complicated genuine emotional contact between the Jewish and German core group members. Both sides were anxious about identifying with the aggressor and the victim within themselves. But after two exhausting days of meeting with Dr. Volkan, the core group members felt that they could now move forward with the process of defining and implementing the aims of their group. They began in earnest to select other German psychiatrists and psychologists for membership in their organization and to identify other influential individuals who could contribute to their cause.

The Third Gathering—February 1998: A Space-Clearing

Three months later, Dr. Volkan arrived for his third "marathon" meeting with the PAKH core group members. In the interim, the group had accomplished much organizational work on the symposium project, but the individual members had also worked hard on emotionally separating mental representations of people and events belonging to the past from those belonging to the present. They were beginning to be able to maintain a "time expansion" (Volkan, 1997b, 1999a). By recognizing in themselves the acute effects of deposited parental images and of their respective chosen traumas relating to the Third Reich period, they could differentiate present Germany from Nazi Germany, while still acknowledging the former as an heir of its past. At this meeting, Dr. Volkan observed that one of the Germans openly wore the Christian symbol of the fish, or *ichthys*, and a Jewish member wore the Star of David. Though neither was consciously aware of it, their choices reflected a new sense that these Jews and Germans could safely come together to do business or to discuss highly emotional issues while openly holding onto their large-group identities.

At the third meeting, the German members were able to speak more openly about their own suffering as a result of association with the Third Reich. The non-Jewish members had been unwilling to tell their own stories because the trauma of the Holocaust for Jews is so great that to speak of non-Jewish Germans' suffering seemed to them a selfish and trivial act. But this very reticence, in turn, had disrupted the communication between the German and Jewish members. Everyone agreed that it was helpful for the representatives of the victimized group to allow the representatives of the victimizer group to speak of their burdens in order to open communication between the two; in fact, it was suggested, allowing the present-day members of the victimizing group to speak might even be a precondition for them to be able to say truly, "We are sorry."

One ethnic German, in fact, had come prepared to speak of his personal history, which, of course, referred directly to events before and during World War II. His was a moving story. His father and two of his friends had opposed the Nazis; one of the friends had killed himself, leaving the impression that he would rather be dead than a Nazi. The member's father had eventually served the Nazis, not as a soldier, but as a food supplier for the German Army; the son carried the impression that his father should have known what was happening. After the war, the father had become a "silent" person. He wished to investigate psychology as a means of understanding human nature, but did not do so. His son had completed his father's task by studying psychology and was now attempting to understand the horror of which his father could not speak. While this participant was talking about his father's silence, the female Jewish member—in whose house the core group was meeting with Dr. Volkan—left the room and returned with a postcard that her father had sent to her five years previously, just before he died. He had signed the postcard "your dumb and silent father." Both German and Jewish fathers had lived silent lives for decades after the Holocaust.

The Fourth Gathering—August 1998: A Revelation

Dr. Volkan's fourth meeting with the PAKH core group took place the day before the symposium. The members showed him the program, printed on yellow paper, and talked about the implications of this color. They had not selected it themselves—the printer had chosen it without consulting them—and the group was somewhat anxious that it evoked memories of the yellow stars that Jews were forced to wear during the Nazi period. But it was too late to change it. One of the ethnic German members lamented, "We can't get away from it [the Nazi past]." Nevertheless, another member recalled that for the Chinese, yellow is a "good" and hopeful color, and the group agreed to look at the inadvertent signifier in this light, rather than dwell on its other possible implications.

It had been decided that they would begin the symposium with six persons—the five core group members and Dr. Volkan—at the podium. Core members, in turn, would spend about five minutes giving the audience some important details about their lives and describing what had first brought them together and why they had worked as a group to organize this event. Following their presentations, Dr. Volkan was to speak about the psychological "anatomy" of their preparations for the symposium. This quite personal beginning significantly set the underlying emotional tone for the entire meeting (Opher-Cohn et al., 2000). What might have been merely an intellectual exercise among historians, psychoanalysts, politicians, and others became—through emotional and moving presentations by Ira Brenner, Annette Streeck-Fischer, and others—a meaningful personal experience of contending with the Third Reich's legacy. Still, as the symposium neared an end, the participants agreed that the question mark of its title persisted: The "end of speechlessness" remained incomplete, an ongoing exercise, a work in progress.

10

The Use of Third Reich Symbols
BY AMERICANS UNAFFECTED BY THE HOLOCAUST

Of course, Germany is not the only home of the neo-Nazi movements to which the last chapter alluded; in the United States, for example, white-supremacist organizations such as Aryan Nations have appropriated the aesthetics of the Third Reich to promote Nazi-like ideals of "racial purity." But neither are Nazi images in the American imagination limited to the demonstrations and publications of racist hate groups. Some of our non-Jewish patients in the United States have also been observed to express their psychopathology or identity issues through Nazi or Holocaust symbols in dreams, fantasies, and delusions. In this chapter, we will examine the cases of four such patients. The first two had siblings with handicaps, and the third, a deformed hand. Because individuals with disabilities were at risk in Nazi Germany, it makes sense that these three individuals contaminated their own internal conflicts, anxieties, and unconscious fantasies and transference manifestations with images of the Third Reich. What is most interesting us here, however, is that none of these three patients were Jewish or German, nor were their families directly affected by the Nazi regime, nor were they or their families involved with neo-Nazi movements. The fourth case reported in this chapter illustrates an even more intriguing phenomenon. In this case, the patient was not only *not* affiliated with any large group affected directly by the Third Reich, but, indeed, had no intimate connection with anyone who would have been in danger in Nazi Germany, such as an individual with a physical or mental disability or a homosexual person.

Pattie and Jane: Siblings with Disabilities and Nazi Expressions

Pattie was 21 years old when she began her analysis with Dr. Volkan. Because the details of Pattie's work with Dr. Volkan have been published elsewhere (Volkan, 1987), the focus here is on her use of Third Reich symbols to express unconscious womb fantasies related to her sibling rivalry and rage against her mother.

Volkan and Ast (1997) have illustrated the commonness of unconscious womb fantasies, as well as their variability (see also Volkan, 1999d). Typically, such fantasies develop in a child when the birth of a younger brother or sister, or the mother's attention to a younger sibling, becomes a traumatic experience for the older child; the older child comes to perceive the younger as an "intruder." When the storyline of the older child's unconscious womb fantasy becomes conscious during analytic work, it generally follows this pattern: Children wish to enter their mother's belly and kill the new fetus. This desire causes a conflict because the wish to kill the fetus (and later the younger sibling) clashes with a fear of losing the mother or her love, or of being punished by the superego. Often children project their aggression onto the fetus and then fear to "enter" the mother's womb—in adulthood, enclosed spaces that symbolize the inside of the mother's belly—because entering the womb means facing a terrifyingly powerful other, the fetus made mighty by the older children's projections. The analytic work is never fully completed until the analyst and the patient reconstruct the pathogenic key unconscious fantasies and make their storyline conscious. Furthermore, patients need to bring these to the transference neurosis to free themselves from the influence of the unconscious fantasies. In Pattie's case, images related to the Third Reich "piggybacked" onto her otherwise typical unconscious womb fantasies.

In the final week of her analysis, Pattie recaptured, for the last time, her dominant pathogenic unconscious womb fantasy. After a session in the late afternoon, Pattie earnestly appealed to Dr. Volkan to let her use his phone. This was a most unusual request; in the course of six and a half years of analysis, Pattie had never requested such a thing. Because no other telephones were available nearby, and because Dr. Volkan did not know the reason for the urgency of Pattie's petition, he gave her permission to use his telephone and left the office while she was talking. This anomalous event had occurred so suddenly, there was no time to discuss it. During the next day's session, however, when the analyst voiced his curiosity, Pattie reported that she had already conducted her own self-analysis about the event, for it had appeared as a day's residue in a dream she had the night following her session. In the dream, she was a princess in a vast mansion. Loudly carousing strangers arrived, forcing Pattie out of the mansion. With the help of a man, she went back to what had been the mansion, but was now just a modest, solidly built stone house. There she encountered a woman with scissors in her hand who tried to cut Pattie's hair. The scissors were sharp at first, but became blunt.

When she awoke, Pattie knew that what she had experienced was a "review dream" (Glover, 1955), an internal review of her whole analysis. The dream reflected her wish to be her father's "princess," as well as her hidden grandiosity at the time she came to analysis, her sibling rivalry globalized. The invaders of the mansion represented her siblings, who, she had felt early in analysis, had displaced her from her rightful elevated place. The man, her analyst, helped her return to the mansion and turn it into a solid house; while the mansion stood for Pattie's former grandiosity, the modest solid house signified her analyzed self-representation. The woman with the scissors represented her mother, who had cut young Pattie's hair more than once, hurting her in the process, and who had cut Pattie's pacifier into pieces when the child was still using it at about age 4 (an expression of Pattie's oral-level fixation).

Upon awakening, Pattie had quickly pieced together this understanding of her dream. As she reported it to Dr. Volkan, however, she began to laugh, as she realized an even deeper significance to the dream: as an expression of a dominant wish that she wanted to satisfy—to become conscious and therefore free of—just before terminating her work with Dr. Volkan. It was only now, Pattie told her analyst, that she realized that she had noticed a pair of scissors in a holder on his desk while she was on the office phone the previous day talking to her sister who formerly had a handicap, who was born when Pattie was two and a half years old. Although this sister developed normally over time, she had early orthopedic problems and as an infant and small child had been required to wear leg braces. The sister's disability had injured Pattie's mother's self-esteem, and the mother had devoted herself to the sister at Pattie's expense. As a result, Pattie had difficulty achieving separation-individuation. She now understood that the woman with scissors in her dream represented not only her punishing mother, but also her own aggressive childhood image; she had wanted to thrust scissors into her mother's womb to kill her sister who had orthopedic problems. Indeed, she had made a point of telling her sister on the phone that she was *alone* in her analyst's office; by being the analyst/mother's only child, she was bringing her dominant pathogenic wish to life by displacing/"killing" her sister. The cutting of her hair and pacifier had been, in her mind, punishments for her murderous rage; because the scissors in the dream were no longer sharp, she could see that she was also successfully taming her own aggression and superego. The narrative represented by the review dream was an old story to her now, and instead of being terrorized by it as in the past, she could now be amused by discerning how she had captured the main points of her total analysis in one event and one dream.

Pattie's final week of work with Dr. Volkan powerfully illustrates her womb fantasy and her childhood experience of murderous rage. What is most interesting here, however, is that because of this murderous rage, before she began her analysis, she had identified with Hitler, despite having no direct connection to the events of the Nazi period in Germany or to any large group affected by those events. Pattie's parents were well-to-do; they belonged to a fancy country club in their community. They were acquainted with other members of the club who were Jewish, and at no time did they express anti-Semitic attitudes to their daughter. But few, if any, of their close friends were Jewish, and no discussion took place in their home of the Third Reich or the Holocaust.

Pattie knew the Nazi regime's policy about persons with disabilities, though she was unaware of either when or how she had learned of it. But from her latency period, or adolescence, she had considered Hitler a "twisted genius" and had been conscious of an identification with the Führer, a fact that sometimes scared her. Thus, when thinking of herself as a Nazi, she would reassure herself that unlike the original Nazis, she would never actually kill. Indeed, she explained this idea to her analyst when they began to work together—in a sense, to reassure him that his life would be spared. Once, as a teenager, Pattie had attacked her mother with a knife. Though she did not harm her mother, Pattie believed deep down that the reassurance that she would not kill needed to be repeated again and again, lest her murderous impulse resurface.

During the first year of her analysis, she had occasionally called Dr. Volkan "Hitler," projecting her own self-image as a murderess onto him. She did not know Dr. Volkan's ethnic background, but often stated her belief that his accent (actually Turkish) was German in origin and that he was a Nazi. Yet the only anti-Semitic remarks that Pattie used during her analysis were directed at her analyst; she accused him of being a "money-grabber" and a "woman-hating Freud." In her transference neurosis, Pattie's personal psychopathology was intermingled with Third Reich images, representing the analyst as both a Nazi and a Jew.

Two years and two months after starting her analysis, Pattie had reported another memorable dream, one that incorporated Third Reich images. In the dream, Pattie was being held captive in a house. A woman wearing what Pattie called "an SM uniform" had tied her to a table. Though "SM" was a slip of the tongue—she meant to say "SS"—Pattie's slip reflected the fact that up to this time, most of Pattie's actual relationships with people around her were in fact sadomasochistic. In the dream, while Pattie lay on the table, the woman wearing the Nazi uniform tore Pattie's body in half. (This part of Pattie's dream is quite similar to the dream, which we mentioned in chapter 9, reported by Dieter Ohlmeier's [1990] male patient.) A man appeared in Pattie's dream, handcuffed the Nazi SS woman, and took her away. Before she left, the woman turned and, apparently having no idea that she had hurt Pattie, said, "You know, I only wanted to love you and give you pleasure."

Not surprisingly, the dream disturbed Pattie. When she entered analysis, Pattie had exhibited a borderline personality organization; the two sections of her body in the dream represented her split self-representation. She told Dr. Volkan with certainty that the Nazi woman in the dream was her mother, onto whose image Pattie also had projected her own murderous self-image; thus she blamed her mother for her own unintegrated self-representation. Because she was lying on the table in the dream as she lay on Dr. Volkan's couch, he was the sadistic mother in the transference, but he was also the man who handcuffed—controlled—the mother. Among various meanings of this dream she generated in analysis, the one that made the strongest impression on Pattie was the realization that her mother's inadequate care had never been a malign design, but an indication that her mother had not known how to love her in the proper fashion. Her mother, who was busy taking care of Pattie's sister who had a handicap, had missed certain mothering functions in her relationship with Pattie.

The next day, Pattie appeared in her session with a new hairstyle. She said that recalling how her mother had tried to help her by cutting her hair, but had only succeeded in pulling it and hurting her, had led her to cut her own hair into a new style. Through the haircut, Pattie symbolically proved her competence in a function at which her mother was deficient. The dream, the analysis of its meaning, and the action taken by Pattie the next day indicated that she had reached a turning point in her analysis.

* * *

Jane, like Pattie, had a sister with a handicap. The first child in the family, this sister had a congenitally malformed lung and probably a heart defect and was never expected to live long. The mother became pregnant again, and Jane was born into an anxious family 15 months after her "deformed" sister. Like Pattie's family, Jane's family was Christian. Jane was born on a farm, and, during her developmental years in a southern state of the United States, the family had no meaningful relationships with people of Jewish faith. As a child, Jane did not study the Nazis or their treatment of European Jews. Neither her father nor other close relatives were involved in the military or support efforts during World War II. Nevertheless, images of the Holocaust played a significant role in the acute psychotic episode Jane experienced when she came to analysis at the age of 21. (Further details of Jane's total treatment have been reported elsewhere [Volkan, 1995].)

When she entered analysis, her inner world was filled with terrifying object images—a devil with her father's face, floating body parts. In time, her analyst learned that among many traumas of her childhood, a key one was the death of her sister who had a handicap. When Jane was 18 months old, her older sister died in her mother's arms on the way to the hospital; the only other passenger in the taxi was Jane herself. Jane subsequently felt that she had lost her mother, who became depressed after the death of her older daughter and who therefore could not mother Jane adequately. Although she retained no conscious memory of her sibling, Jane suffered throughout her childhood from a kind of survivor guilt, no doubt reflecting her mother's complicated grief, depression, and frequent references to the child she had lost. But Jane was not aware of this fact until, in the course of therapeutic regression, she came to recognize her attempted identification with her sister who had a deformity. More than once, on Dr. Volkan's couch, she distorted her limbs so as to look deformed and crippled.

Jane was an artist, and during the initial phase of her analysis, when her treatment reactivated memories and affects of her childhood, as well as the images of her sister kept alive in her parents' minds, she obsessively painted dozens of pictures of Holocaust victims. Jane, who was born in 1943, might have seen images of Holocaust survivors in newspapers or magazines while growing up or as an adult, although she had no conscious recollection of having done so. The Holocaust victims in her art stood as representations of her sister who had a deformity and corresponding representations of herself as one psychologically undernourished because of inadequate mothering. She stopped this type of painting as she got well.

Ricky: Hitler's "Right Arm"

Like Pattie's and Jane's families, the family of our third case had no direct connection with the Third Reich or its aftermath. Ricky, 18 years old when he entered treatment, had a disability; he had been born with small digits on his right hand and right foot. His mother had marked each of his birthdays, beginning with the fourth, by giving him a wedding ring too large for his fingers. Through this bizarre behavior, Ricky's mother constantly denied that her son had a handicap, while at the same time reminding her son how ashamed she was of his "deformity." The message was that the son should deny having a handicap, as his mother attempted to do; the deformity became a psychological "secret" that they shared. Furthermore, this behavior was only one of many that reflected the mother's inability to help her son achieve sound reality-testing or healthy individuation. It is little wonder that the boy, though brilliant, grew up to become schizophrenic.

As a teenager, instead of studying the usual subjects in school, Ricky read everything he could find on Nazi history. He became very knowledgeable on the subject indeed; if one asked him what had happened on a certain date in the Third Reich, he could recite the events of that date in detail. Of all the Nazis that Ricky studied, Joseph Goebbels was of special interest to him. It should be recalled that Goebbels had a clubfoot, which had kept him out of service in World War I. Named propaganda minister in 1933, Goebbels had complete control over the press, radio, and even cinema and theater. Highly intelligent and devoted to Hitler, Goebbels was not only instrumental in popularizing National Socialism in Germany and abroad, but also in helping Hitler to remain in power. Because of his clubfoot, Goebbels was an eminently suitable object-image for Ricky's identification. Like Goebbels, he could spread untruth: For Ricky, the untruth that he was not "deformed." Furthermore, Ricky saw Goebbels as Hitler's strong "right arm"; identifying with Goebbels, Ricky created, albeit in a psychotic fashion, a nondeformed arm and hand. He called his mother "Hitler" and submitted himself to her as he thought Goebbels would have submitted to the Führer, together propagating the idea that he had no physical disability. Since he gave himself as a "strong arm" (a phallic symbol) to his mother, Ricky also made her into a "phallic mother." Walking, as he often did, in a rigid fashion imitative of a Nazi soldier's "goose-stepping," he turned his whole body, symbolically, into an erect penis. By submitting to his mother, he unconsciously protected himself from aggressive attack, mutilation, or castration; because his mother would possess her own "phallus" in him, she would not castrate him.

Ricky had sensed that behind her denial of his disability, his mother was ashamed of him. A narcissistic affront to her self-esteem, she had wished that he did not exist. Through his delusional identification with Goebbels, who became the strong "right arm" of the Führer despite his clubfoot, Ricky protected himself against being murdered by Nazis, his mental representation of the mother who wished him dead.

Claire: Trapped in a Nazi "Anal Prison"

Claire was a 53-year-old divorcée with two grown children when she entered analysis for chronic depression, muscular aches and pains, and severe constipation. Several years earlier, she had undergone surgical repair of a prolapsed rectum. A talented poet, she also complained of being singularly unproductive in her work for many months because she spent most of her time practicing obsessional rituals. She had an extensive psychiatric history, including six months as an inpatient in her early 20s after an abortive suicide attempt. She had two siblings, neither of whom had a disability, and her own body was "normal" as well. In the initial interview, she reported that she had been plagued by what she called recurrent "concentration camp dreams" between the ages of 30 and 40. In these dreams, she would search for means of escape, but to no avail, and she would awaken in a panicked state. In the third year of her analysis with Dr. Greer, these dreams began to recur. Before we present some of these manifestations of Third Reich images, however, let us briefly review her developmental history.

For the first two years of Claire's life, she was raised by her maternal grandmother because her own mother was too severely incapacitated by postpartum depression to care for her. Her father, a veteran of World War II, was in military service at that time in the European theater, but he was apparently not particularly traumatized by the experience in any way that would subsequently affect his daughter. When Claire was a very small child, we suspect that one or both of her parents gave her enemas, because she reported that this was a routine practice with her younger sister. Moreover, as an adult, she gave herself enemas and experienced an intense urge to be given an enema in sexual foreplay. When her transference neurosis was fully developed, she even asked Dr. Greer to give her enemas—another indication that she was probably given enemas as a child. The only enema that she could consciously recall having received had been administered by a nurse, in the presence of her mother, after she was hospitalized at age 6 for constipation. The child's perception of this event was that her "amused" mother—not the nurse, significantly—aggressively intruded her body and stole her insides.

Another trauma occurred when Claire was 12 years old, in the midst of the obligatory adolescent regression (Blos, 1979) in which preoedipal and oedipal images and conflicts are revivified and worked through. At this time, her alcoholic father came to her bed and rubbed her genitals as her mother watched. Claire was emaciated and weak when this occurred, due to a severe illness that had nearly killed her. Claire adapted to these traumas by reaching "up," developmentally (Boyer, 1983, 1999; Volkan, 1976), to an anal fixation in order to escape the oral-level trauma primarily caused by her mother, and by moving "down," regressively, to an anal fixation in order to escape the oedipal-level trauma primarily caused by her father. Thus, in a sense, she grew up in an "anal prison" and remained there for the rest of her life.

As an adult, Claire went to see three therapists, all of whom, unfortunately, were poorly trained, and who ended up behaving like her parents. Actualizing her expectation that there was no escape from her "anal prison" by replaying the roles of her invading parents in transference, two of them became sexually involved with Claire, and the third socialized with her. Desperate and aware that this was perhaps her last chance to work through her emotional difficulties, Claire began treatment with Dr. Greer.

During the first eight months of her third year of treatment, Claire reported a series of dreams incorporating images of the Third Reich. In the first of these, she worked as a servant in a luxurious house where the lampshades were made out of human skin. This recalled to her the cowhide lampshades in a favorite vacation resort that she and her parents visited when she was a child, suggesting that she was beginning to acknowledge her childhood environment as psychologically "murderous." In another dream, she tried to seduce a Nazi guard so that a woman, whom Claire believed to represent herself, could escape. The woman was captured and summarily executed. Here, Claire used Nazi symbols to repeat her past trauma at the hands of her father (in the transference, Dr. Greer). She was either going to seduce him and repeat the trauma under her control, or be killed by him as a representative of her own projected murderous rage condensed with her father's aggression toward her. In yet another dream that included a Third Reich motif, she was being herded to a platform where she was to board a boxcar that would take her to a camp. She thought she might try to break away from the group but knew that the guards would quickly recapture her. She then thought that perhaps she could crawl under the boxcar, hold onto the undercarriage of the train, and drop off onto the tracks after the train was underway—but realized that guard dogs would sniff her out. The day's residue for this dream included affect-laden childhood memories—induced by seeing the story of a girl with a cochlear implant on the cover of a magazine in Dr. Greer's office—of being slapped so hard by her father that it caused hearing loss; the memory of paternal abuse was condensed with the image of Nazi threat in her dream. On still another occasion, Claire dreamed of a column of people, guarded on both sides by Nazis, being marched off to a "shower" where, she knew, they would all be gassed. She realized that if she did not steal away quietly from the group, her fate would be sealed. The next night, she dreamed of seeing an analyst who wore his hair like Hitler's, from whom she hid in a room where guards came searching for her. Dr. Greer explained to Claire that via transference, her dream reflected that she perceived her childhood environment as a concentration camp where she had been the victim of "soul murder" (Shengold, 1989).

During the time period in which Claire reported such dreams, she symbolically turned Dr. Greer's office into an "anal prison." She habitually arrived for her sessions early enough to spend some time in the lavatory next to the waiting room, where she would inspect the toilet and toilet tissues for any remains of fecal matter. In her sessions, she spoke at length about her activities in "Dr. Greer's bathroom," as she called it. Eventually, Claire made a symbolic toilet of the couch; her sessions were filled with direct and indirect references to her attachment to or dread of receiving enemas and her desire to produce or to withhold her feces. She became preoccupied with her own bowel movements and grew intensely sensitive to the odors associated with anal activities. Sometimes she was concerned that she smelled badly and sometimes fantasized that Dr. Greer passed gas during her sessions. She was paralyzed with anal ambivalence.

By actualizing her "anal prison" in the space where she worked through her Nazi-infused dreams, Claire, in a sense, brought to life her childhood fixation at the anal phase *through* Nazi images and expressions. The Nazi symbols she used primarily represented her anal rage: She, as a Nazi, could explode and kill others; or, others, on whom she projected her anal sadism, could kill her. Gradually, the therapeutically progressive aspects of her activities and associations came into focus. Claire wanted to "kill" her anally fixated, Nazi-identified self and the object-images that played a role in her fixation. If she "killed" that part of herself, however, her identification with the Nazis would remain; she would be a murderer. Underlying this wish was the desire to escape her "anal prison" so that she could bring her oral and oedipal traumas to the transference neurosis—that is, so that she could re-experience being the baby with a depressed mother and the child whose genitals were invaded by her father. Only by working through the conflicts that caused her anal fixation could she hope to get fully well. But Claire had a serious dilemma. Because her pathogenic past with her parents had been repeated in reality with dangerous individuals calling themselves therapists, she displayed great resistance to leaving her "anal prison" and moving on to oral and phallic areas of her life with Dr. Greer, for fear that he, too, would violate her. It is beyond our topic here to report further on Claire's treatment, but we can report that Claire has, happily, been able to move beyond her "anal prison" and to terminate her analysis.

Part 3
THERAPEUTIC CONSIDERATIONS

11

Different Cases, DIFFERENT APPROACHES

THE ABUNDANT USE OF NAZI AND HOLOCAUST SYMBOLS and unconscious fantasies by patients in no way directly affected by the Third Reich reflects the degree to which the Holocaust's cataclysmic recasting of human history (Moses, 1993) has wrought a change in *internalized* human history as well. Before considering the technical issues involved in treating the consequences of that change, however, we wish to emphasize that we belong to that group of clinicians who, as Peter Giovacchini (2000) writes, "have roamed freely in the realms of object relations but have not forsaken thinking in terms of intrapsychic forces conflicting with each other, which, in some circles, has become politically incorrect" (p. 87). We do not regard as properly psychoanalytic any therapeutic process that depends on ideas that are more philosophical than clinical, or that fails to take into account intrapsychic unconscious factors, such as the influence of unconscious fantasies, mental conflicts, defenses, resistances, and transference neuroses. We consider ourselves in the mainstream of psychoanalysis.

Two Categories of "Unaffected" Individuals: Symbolic and Protosymbolic

Pattie, Jane, Ricky, and Claire were neither directly affected by the Nazi regime, nor were they offspring of people who were directly affected, yet they still used Holocaust images, Nazi images, or both to express some of their internal processes. Such "unaffected individuals" may usefully be divided into two categories:

In the first category are *those who have cohesive core identities* but unconsciously perceive similarities between Nazi expressions and images and their own drive expressions and self- and object-images. These individuals deploy Nazi- and victim-images as *symbols*, which have, as Burness Moore and Bernard Fine (1990) state, "a conscious manifest form but also latently [represent] unconscious mental content, and the relationship between the symbol and its referent is not arbitrary but is based on, for example, some perceived similarity or analogy: a house might represent the human body or a tower represent the penis" (p. 191).

Those who have deficiencies in their identity formations and who fill in the cracks in their identities with "cement" made of victim- or Nazi-images belong to the second category of unaffected individuals. These people utilize Third Reich-related images as *protosymbols*, which Heinz Werner and Bernard Kaplan (1963) define as structures that "directly 'present' a meaning rather than 'represent' it" (p. 16). On the surface, protosymbols are often undistinguishable from symbols, but they lack "the *intentional* act by which a vehicular form is taken to represent a referent. Nevertheless, protosymbols are extremely important in the genetic process of symbolization: protosymbols may be transformed into true symbols by progressive differentiation of vehicle and referential meaning; true symbols may regress to protosymbols through dedifferentiation of vehicle and referent" (pp. 16–17). People who use protosymbols have "unthinkable" experiences and anxieties—that is, mental content is expressed in a concrete, dramatic *presentation* rather than in abstract, verbal *representation*. As long as such protosymbolic means of communication prevail in treatment, the patient's mental content cannot be "thought about," but only repetitively and concretely re-experienced. As Susan Deri (1978) notes, "Symbolization *is* communication across a boundary" (p. 48); in these individuals, there is, as yet, no well-delineated inner space that is ordinarily denoted as "the mind." The transition from symbiosis to separation, from the concrete to the abstract, from the protosymbolic to the symbolic, is accompanied by the gradual development of a differentiated mental space in which mental content can be thought about, as well as experienced.

Claire, despite her severe neurosis and anal character (Abraham, 1949), did not have gaps or cracks in her core identity; her self-representation was cohesive. She unconsciously sensed a resonance, however, between Nazi aggression and her experience of her own anal sadistic aggression combined with her parents' aggression toward her. Individuals in the first category, such as Claire, deploy Nazi or Holocaust symbols very much as anyone might use an image of a historical event as a true symbol. Recently, for instance, an American man dreamed of the terrorist Osama bin Laden to symbolize his murderous self-image. Another American—a woman who, as a child, was emotionally starved—associated herself with a malnourished Biafran girl she had seen on the television news, and she became preoccupied with efforts to eradicate hunger in Biafra, even though she did not even know exactly where it was located. Claire easily understood that Nazi- and victim-symbols were true symbols standing for aggressive drive expressions and self- and object-images from her traumatic childhood. When she reported the dream of being marched off to the shower, she could, with her therapist's help, freely associate from the dream to events that had left her in an "anal prison." Her reference to being gassed like a Jewish victim reflected her own anal rage—which, condensed with her parents' rage toward her, had been projected onto the image of a Nazi murderer. She also easily associated toward the belief that through enemas, her mother had tried to murder her soul (Shengold, 1989). Furthermore, taking a shower signified her reaction formation; she was cleansing her self-representation of both her anal rage and her parents' rage. Thus Claire's use of Nazi symbols did not need to be a primary focus of her treatment; once her developing transference neurosis activated the symbols, the therapy focused on the transference neurosis itself, and the meaning of the symbols could simply be interpreted. For patients like Claire, the symbol itself does not necessarily induce great affective response; the affect surfaces once what the symbol represents is uncovered. (There is one exception to this "rule": The symbol itself induces great affect for neurotic-level individuals when it becomes a phobic object. In order not to experience the affect, the phobic patient avoids the symbolic object; for example, Jacob's "selective blindness" toward the word *exit*. For Jacob, seeing the word *exit* paradoxically recreated horrible affect relating to the fact that there was no exit for Jews from the Holocaust. [See chapter 5.])

Ricky, on the other hand, belonged to the second category of unaffected individuals: those who use Nazi images to patch up their damaged core identities. Individuals in this category often exhibit omnipotent sadism, which may be expressed outwardly. Sometimes, the sadism turns on part of oneself, since the "Nazi" and the "Jewish" images may coexist, in a split fashion, within such individuals. We suspect that many unaffected individuals in the United States who have become neo-Nazis are filling deficiencies in their identity formations with Nazi images. In other patients, however, the victim image may be dominant, attracting and collecting victimizers in the environment like a magnet.

For people who belong to this second category, the distance between the representing element and what is represented intermingle. The "as if" aspect of the Nazi symbol disappears; in the individual's mind the protosymbol *is* what it is supposed to *represent*. Ricky, as was discussed earlier, experienced his mother as Hitler and his corresponding self-image as Goebbels. Nazi images induced great emotion for him, because there was little or no distance between them and what they stood for. The patient in the second category may even experience the analyst in the transference as a protosymbol—the analyst *is* a Nazi or *is* a Jewish victim. In his first session, for example, Ricky smacked his lips together in a peculiar way; when Dr. Volkan asked him what he was doing, Ricky reported that he was "tasting" the analyst like a mouthful of wine to see whether he was "a good German or a bad German." There was no "as if" in his transference with Dr. Volkan; the analyst *was* German, and Ricky's only question was about his allegiance. Under such conditions, the analyst and the patient need to "play" with the protosymbols *within the therapeutic space* until they become true symbols. It then becomes possible to examine and work through the symbols' multiple meanings, their close associations with unconscious fantasies, and, most important, their connections with the individual's core identity problems.

To summarize, then, first-category unaffected persons do not present any special therapeutic difficulties, particularly if neither the analyst nor the analyst's ancestors were directly affected by the Third Reich. Unaffected individuals in the second category, however, are like directly affected persons, insofar as Nazi-related images are integral parts of the core identities of both. Accordingly, the technical aspects of treating directly affected individuals that will be outlined next are also applicable to treating second-category unaffected individuals.

Obstacles to Treatment: "Affected" Individuals with "Mild" Cases

From the beginning of this project, we have recognized that not every descendant of parents or grandparents traumatized during the Third Reich exhibits psychopathology. Although all directly affected descendants' identities are likely reservoirs for Nazi-related deposited images, associated affects, unconscious fantasies, and chosen trauma *regardless of whether their core identities are cohesive*, people deploy those deposited images in different ways. Indeed, some such individuals may possess a high level of adaptive capacity and may develop creative sublimations; these people are among the ranks of our most prominent and admired scholars, artists, and humanitarians—including, as we saw in chapters 8 and 9, our psychoanalytic colleagues. Their situation is not unlike that of "replacement children." All such children's core identities contain parents' or caretakers' images of the dead siblings or other relatives for whom they function as "replacements." Less adaptive replacement children will have trouble integrating their own self-images with the deposited images of the dead relatives; for these children, the deposited images may act like irritating "foreign objects" within their self-representations. Replacement children with high intelligence and adaptive capacity will not be injured by the deposited images if they can match their activities and mental products with those that the parents or other caregivers expect from the now-idealized deposited image. As Brenner (1991) observes, however, the psychological legacy of the Nazi regime "manifests itself in a variety of forms and presents an ongoing challenge in therapy" (p. 98) for descendants of those who lived under the Third Reich.

In what we are calling *mild cases*, affected descendants' self-representations assimilate, to a great extent, their ancestors' deposited images relating to the historical trauma, and affects related to these images are substantially tamed. For practical purposes, mild-case patients have cohesive identities. Nazi/victimizer and Jewish/victim images in their unconscious fantasies are not contaminated with omnipotent sadism or masochism. And when the meanings of their unconscious fantasies and related projections, introjections, displacements, splittings, denial, reaction formations, and isolation mechanisms are interpreted, mild-case patients easily understand the deposited images' influence on their identities.

Ira Brenner (1988, 1991) reports the case of a Jewish woman patient, the child of a Holocaust survivor, who echoed the concerns about parenthood that arose in the cases of Uta and Leo, whose cases were reviewed in chapters 6 and 7. Brenner's patient sought treatment with a specific question in mind: She wanted to know whether she should have a baby. After some hesitation, the patient revealed that her boyfriend was German. His father had been in Warsaw during World War II, and she sometimes wondered what her boyfriend's family had done during the Nazi period:

> Although she insisted spontaneously that her boyfriend was "innocent" because he was born after the war, the prospect of carrying around the grandchild of a Nazi in her womb was clearly a major issue to her. The life and death struggle between German and Jew was being enacted in the form of an unconscious "selection," as she tried to enlist the doctor's help in making a medical decision—if she should give life to such a child. (p. 98)

Brenner adds that this patient had unconsciously cast her psychiatrist in the role of an SS doctor on the arrival platform at Auschwitz by asking him to decide whether a life was worth saving. Whether this patient's case should be considered "mild" would depend on her ability to respond positively to this interpretation, as well as on the intensity of affect invested in her images of Nazis and victims. If she were a mild case, the therapist would only need to interpret, at the therapeutically correct time, what is relevant and what unconscious, and the patient would finally make up her own mind about marrying a German.

In mild cases, treating the descendants of those who lived under the Third Reich is not *fundamentally* different than the analysis of many patients of the first category of unaffected persons outlined earlier in this chapter. For such mild cases, the accepted, time-tested "rules and regulations" of psychoanalytic methodology all apply to the task of raising to the surface Holocaust- and other Nazi-related unconscious fantasies, assigning conscious storylines to them, and working through the conflicts they create. In the long run, the therapeutic focus rests on identity issues, as the affected offspring learn more about the deposited images and identifications and the influence of these on the offspring's identities. Several potential obstacles to this work, however, are unique to the treatment of all directly affected persons, whether they are affiliated with the "victim" group or the "victimizer" group.

First, the work of making conscious what has been unconscious necessarily raises "unacceptable" feelings, such as pain, guilt, shame, and entitlement, and brings to consciousness identification with murderous or helpless individuals—unpleasant feelings and thoughts of which the patient will resist becoming aware.

Sheldon Roth (1993) and Rafael Moses (1993) both provide us with lists of barriers to Holocaust awareness among Jewish patients, including marked anxiety over separation and loss; unwillingness to report "unacceptable" sadomasochistic wishes; fear of passivity and helplessness; derivations of survivor guilt; a sense of shame, sense of entitlement, or both; and an inability to mourn or difficulty in taming aggression and mourning. German patients, on the other hand, may resist recognizing identification with the Nazis or may fear finding something "monstrous" within themselves, like Anna Maria Jokl's (1997) patient who envisioned himself as a gigantic beast, isolated in a dark cave, that would kill the women whose embraces he desired. At the same time, ethnic German patients may fear generational discontinuity if they dis-identify with their ancestors. They may also trivialize their trauma, since it cannot compare to the trauma shared by the victimized group, and they may envy other large groups that do not share such a shameful history (Appy, 1993).

To these findings, we need to add another observation important for treating such patients. It is especially difficult for patients from chosen trauma-evolving groups—whether they come from the victim- or the victimizer-group—to deal with the derivatives of their aggressive drives. Those who exhibit the influence of deposited images, identifications, and history-related unconscious fantasies may unconsciously connect their own sense and expression of aggression with the horrible acts of history. If they are going to get well, these patients need to learn how to feel and express "normal" anger—even to enjoy it, once they finally accept that "normal" anger does not kill.

Special Countertransference Problems

In some patients whose conflicts have become pathogenically contaminated with the mental images of their large group's history, it is difficult, if not impossible, to analyze more routine preoedipal and oedipal conflicts without fully taking this image into account. Such contaminated conflicts are like tar on sand: One cannot see the sand (the individual's internal processes) until one removes the tar (the legacy of the large group's history that has leached into those processes and contaminated them). When the contaminant is removed through therapeutic work, more usual developmental conflicts appear clearly and working through them becomes more routine. Because psychoanalysts are not typically trained to recognize the potential influence of such large-group historical contaminants in their analyzands' expressions, however, the influence of these remains largely unanalyzed. Analysts may also fail to recognize the derivatives of such historical material in their patients' internalized object relations, symptoms, character traits, and transference manifestations because the analysts themselves may belong to a traumatized or aggressor large group and may therefore maintain unanalyzed defenses that prevent them from being aware of such conflicts within themselves. The patient and the analyst may then unconsciously collude to keep the threatening material out of the analysis.

Harold Blum's (1985) study of a Jewish patient who came to him for reanalysis illustrates the extent to which mutual resistances may prevail when both analyst and analyzand belong to the same traumatized large group. The patient's first analyst, who was also Jewish, failed to "hear" their group's shared trauma in his analyzand's material; in consequence, mutually sanctioned silence and denial pervaded the entire analytic experience, leaving unanalyzed residues of the Holocaust in the analyzand's symptoms. Blum writes, "Although the patient and his last analyst were both born in Europe and were both Jewish, neither one discussed the experience of debasing bigotry, the war, emigration, being a refugee, social-cultural upheaval, separation from family and friends and cultural shock. For years they spoke to each other without mention of each other's accent or why they were meeting in an American rather than a European office" (p. 898). There was, he continues, "a double standard in analysis. Freedom of thought and expression were compromised by tacit cues that some areas were off limits and should remain shrouded in silence. This repetition of the 'conspiracy of silence' (and the suffering in silence of the family) was maintained by depriving memory of emotional meaning, and skillful displacement of discussion" (p. 899).

Such shared resistances are not limited, of course, to Third Reich–related cases; analysts observe them even in those considered "routine" in the States. In an exemplary case, the analyzand was a man from the American South who entered analysis with a newcomer from the North. He assumed that the Northern analyst held Southerners and their cultural heritage in contempt and imagined that his analyst secretly considered him a social and intellectual inferior. "You Northerners," railed the patient, "think you are so damned superior to us benighted Southerners." His father was a devout Southern Baptist whose own grandfather had been killed in the Civil War and whose parents were brought up during the Reconstruction era. The father had unconsciously transmitted to his son the humiliated self-image passed to him by the ancestors who had been defeated by the "Yankees." The patient's father had never directly spoken of this sense of humiliation, yet it had often been communicated to the analyzand indirectly. For example, just before a trip to the North to visit his prospective son-in-law's parents, the father was heard to say, "If those damn Yankees high hat me, I'll walk out." Both the father's and son's identities, then, included aspects of their ancestors' humiliated self-image, together with defenses against it. Identifying with the traumatized image of his defeated and humiliated ancestors, the patient's eyes would moisten as he envisaged dispirited Confederate soldiers, heads shamefully bowed, making the long trek back to their homes. He was, perhaps, engaged in an attempted mourning of the losses incurred by his large group more than a hundred years earlier: losses so massive that the large group was unable to mourn them at that time. In a sense, the wretched souls of his ancestors, unable to find rest from their trauma, occupied this man's internal world; essentially, his core identity, large-group regional identity (Southern), and national identity (American) had become intertwined. Such historical references may usefully be thought of as a prism through which more typical psychosexual conflicts, such as those associated with the oedipal complex, may pass.

Under certain circumstances, then, analysts may—resisting awareness of the influence of the group's shared trauma on their own internal world—become utterly oblivious to the derivative expressions of these in their patients' associations and behavior. Such analyst-supported resistance is now gradually becoming recognized even in Germany as a crucial therapeutic issue. In the early 1960s, while treating an ethnic German analyzand and a Jewish analyzand, German Jewish analyst Anna Maria Jokl left for Israel without completing the two patients' analytic work, but it was not until the mid-1990s that she was able to piece together and report the complex influences of their large-group identities on the scene of analysis (Jokl, 1997). German psychoanalysts Ilse Grubrich-Simitis (1979), Anita Eckstaedt (1989), and Annette Streeck-Fischer (1999) have explored the difficulties of hearing and having empathy with Nazi-related influences in their German and Jewish patients. Eckstaedt, indeed, has brought overdue attention to the trauma that ethnic Germans themselves experienced during the Third Reich and to the influences of that trauma on the self-conception of contemporary Germans.

At this point, it should go without saying that we firmly believe that analysts and therapists treating patients with unconscious fantasies concerning the Holocaust and Third Reich (or other massive shared traumas) need to be fully conversant with the relevant history. When Dr. Ast revealed that she had been reading about Jenish history and language, Uta was not merely grateful for her analyst's attention; it was only then that "Jenishness" became "real" for Uta as something that existed in the world, even though it had existed within her all along. Thus verbalizing aspects of the large-group history, at appropriate moments, can be a valuable technical maneuver to verify the patient's large-group identity and its symbolic elements. Similarly, Ilse Grubrich-Simitis (1979) underscores the need, in psychoanalytic treatment of the second generation of victims of persecution, to explore the main facts of what actually happened to the parents in order to release patients from "remembering through actions."

Those treating patients with deposited Nazi images should also understand the nature of the relationship between individual and large-group identities, especially the chosen trauma component of the latter (Volkan 1997b, 1999a, 1999b)—another significant form of resistance that has been less well-considered in the clinical literature (although not entirely ignored: see Brenner, 1991). Because consciously and unconsciously held "victim" or "victimizer" images forge bonds between various individuals in their large group (see also chapter 4), patients may unconsciously perceive breaking the silence surrounding the psychological influence of such images of past shared trauma as a threat to their large-group identity. In order to give up this strong resistance, patients need to reach the conclusion that they can still belong to their large group without experiencing the malignant influence of unconscious fantasies related to the historical trauma the group has collectively experienced. As Uta learned, a person does not need to remove the legacy of her people's past from her core identity in order to get well.

Obstacles to Treatment: "Affected" Individuals with "Difficult" Cases

Difficult cases present the psychotherapist or psychoanalyst with a different situation entirely, differing from mild ones in four interrelated areas: First, difficult patients' self-representations and corresponding object-representations are not integrated, though they may possess cohesive aspects of self- and internalized objects to some degree. Second, in difficult patients' unconscious fantasies, "victim" and "victimizer" images are invested with extreme sadism and masochism. Third, their external symbols expressing deposited images, unconscious fantasies, and identifications are experienced as protosymbols. Fourth, individuals do not respond to interpretations positively until they learn to relate to these protosymbols as symbols and tame the affects attached to these. That is, difficult patients' unconscious fantasies are "actualized"—or, in Bergmann's (1982) and Kogan's (2000) term, "concretized." When the derivatives of their fantasies' storylines are reactivated in daily life or in transference, these patients may not be able to tell where fantasy ends and reality begins. Though at one level they may appear to be living normal or neurotic adult lives (a reflection of the parts of their self-representations that are integrated), at another, such individuals' internal worlds are populated with Hitlers or other Nazi protosymbols split from images of victims awaiting annihilation, also experienced as protosymbols (a reflection of the unintegrated aspects of their self-representations): These are people living in two worlds. Before we outline the technical issues relevant to such cases, here is a brief example of a Third Reich–related "difficult" case.

After losing her parents when she was a young adult, Rebecca, the only child of Holocaust survivors, began to keep dozens of cats in her apartment. She spent her energy taking care of the animals, at the expense of her freedom to have a normal social life or to travel. Although Rebecca left home to work in an office, where she was perceived as an efficient and responsible employee, she and her pets were virtually imprisoned in her apartment the rest of the time. One way to understand her behavior is to think of Rebecca as a reservoir for images belonging to parents who were unable to mourn for their relatives killed in the Holocaust. Rebecca was unconsciously given the task of resolving the parental inability to mourn; her response was to develop an unconscious fantasy "reincarnating" the dead relatives in her protosymbolic relationship to her pets.

When four of her cats died together suddenly, she, like her parents, could not mourn her relatives' death, and instead became acutely depressed.

Associating to the names she had given her pets, Rebecca quickly revealed that her cats represented not only her deceased parents, but also many dead aunts, uncles, and other relatives whom she had never known. This behavior is not idiosyncratic; the use of pets or even plants to "reincarnate" relatives who were victims of the Nazis has been well documented. For example, Judith Kestenberg (1989) reports the case of a woman who was attached to her cow and her plants, "with which she consciously conversed as if they were her parents" (p. 391); these inanimate and "living linking objects" (Volkan, 1981, pp. 316–351) connected her, as a survivor, to those who were lost during the Holocaust. Rebecca had externalized onto the cats the mental representations of lost relatives deposited in her by her parents, using the animals primarily as protosymbols. She put the animals, as well as herself, in a "prison," as her parents and relatives had been imprisoned in Nazi camps. Understanding this obvious significance of Rebecca's cats is sufficient to demonstrate the existence of transgenerational transmission, but—unlike in the treatment of "mild" cases—the therapist's proper interpretation is not sufficient for a patient like Rebecca to rid herself of the Third Reich–related influences on her psyche. Rebecca did not respond to the animals *as if* they represented her dead relatives; rather, in her experience, the animals *were* her dead relatives.

When she became depressed after the four animals' deaths, she re-experienced losing her parents and relatives, whose deaths she was unable to mourn properly. And complicating her psychopathology was the fact that Rebecca's protosymbolic relationship to the cats was imbued with extreme sadism and masochism. Overtly, Rebecca loved her cats and devoted her life to them, even to self-sacrificing excess; covertly, though, she was sadistic toward them. In time, Rebecca revealed that the four cats had died because she had put them in a tightly covered box. Consciously, she believed that being in the dark would calm the animals, but, of course, the animals had died because of the heat and lack of air inside the box. In a sense, Rebecca had "gassed" the cats; Rebecca was acting under the influence of another large-group history-related unconscious fantasy that she had developed. Over time, she related other "accidents" in which animals died or at least became severely ill. Surely, Rebecca, like her parents, did not know how to mourn properly; killing the cats was also probably part of an unsuccessful attempt to initiate a process of mourning the dead relatives, since that process involves mourners withdrawing ("killing") their investment in the lost object.

Under her inability to mourn, however, lay the main conflict within her unintegrated core identity: Beneath a surface competence, her self-image as a helpless Jew clashed constantly with her self-image as a sadistic Nazi murderer; her history-related unconscious fantasies made her both a "repairer" and a "destroyer." Her parents had deposited into her these images of helpless victims, as well as of sadistic victimizers, and had prevented her from developing an integrated and cohesive core identity. At home, away from strangers' eyes, Rebecca's parents exhibited their Nazi-tattooed arms to the little child and regularly declared themselves helpless to manage even routine tasks of everyday life. When their child tried to express her own autonomy, however, the parents would become enraged and crush the little girl's enthusiasm. Her inadequate mother had interfered again and again in her daughter's attempts to develop her own individuality; living with helpless rage, Rebecca had developed the unconscious fantasy that she was a Nazi and could avenge herself on her Jewish parents. Throughout her adult life, an identification with Dr. Josef Mengele, the "Angel of Death" at Birkenau and Auschwitz, periodically came to her consciousness, though each time she quickly shook off such thoughts. As a Jew, this patient saw herself as an ultimate sufferer, doomed to live in a prison. Secretly, as a Nazi, she saw herself as an ultimate torturer, doomed to be a killer. In both scenarios, she experienced herself as omnipotent; in her unconscious fantasies, she was both the savior of her victimized relatives and an "angel of death." The cats, primarily as protosymbols, *were* victims to be saved or to be killed.

Rebecca's behavior recalls certain expressions of Leo's and Uta's self-concepts. Leo, who had identified with his mother's ambition and his father's intellectual pursuits, was an accomplished professional and intellectual himself. Nevertheless, he lived a double life as Rebecca did, one in public (which depended upon his integrated self-representation) and one internally and secretly experienced (which mainly expressed his unintegrated self- and object-images). After Leo realized that he had not "killed" Dr. Greer and returned to treatment, he began within a year to experience his former Jewish/victim and Nazi/murderer protosymbols as symbols. When on the way to recovery, Leo recalled his internal life as both a victim (covert) and a Nazi (overt) and declared that he had been unable to visit his mother when she was terminally ill because his fantasy of being a Nazi/murderer was a reality for him; he believed that he would actually kill his mother if he visited her, and symbolically killing her or her representation would thus be beyond reach. Leo had to come to understand that fantasizing is not equivalent to doing (Grubrich-Simitis, 1979). Uta, who also had an unintegrated core identity, was unlike Rebecca and Leo in that she had invested the split parts of her self-representation with less sadism and masochism. As she once tried to become infected with AIDS in order to kill her Aryan boyfriend and at least once behaved masochistically by provoking one of her boyfriends to hit her, Uta's case can be construed as lying somewhere between "mild" and "difficult" cases, as we have outlined them in this chapter. She fantasized that she could kill or be killed, but did not attempt to kill in reality. By contrast, the internal worlds of patients like Leo and Rebecca can best be understood if they are seen as suffering from a form of "malignant narcissistic personality organization" (Kernberg, 1975; Volkan and Ast, 1994).

Malignant Narcissim: The Common Bond of "Difficult" Cases

Before focusing on its malignant forms, let us review the current understanding of the internal worlds of persons with routine narcissistic personality organization. Otto Kernberg (1970, 1975) proposed that integration of the internalized self- and object-images occurs in the narcissistic personality at a level of development in which ego boundaries have already become stable. At this point, he argues, there is "a fusion of ideal self, ideal object, and actual self-images as a defense against an intolerable reality in the interpersonal realm, with a concomitant devaluation and destruction of object images as well as of external objects" (p. 53). The fusion of the ideal self-, ideal object-, and actual self-images creates a *grandiose self*, which is split off from the devalued aspects of the personality.

The three elements that create the grandiose self are configured in the following way: The *real self* is created because the mother or other caretaker sees something special in the child and reinforces it; being special is real for the child. But the caretaker who perceives the child as special is also depriving or overindulging—in a word, frustrating. Thus the child develops an *ideal self* that is endowed with power, beauty, and superiority: a compensation for the frustration of rage and envy at the oral level. The *ideal object* is the fantasized image of a limitlessly providing caretaker. Unacceptable aspects of the real self and devalued external object-images are split off from the grandiose self in a combination sometimes called the *hungry self* (Volkan and Ast, 1994).

The behavior patterns of a person with a narcissistic personality organization primarily reflect the internal relationships between the split grandiose and hungry selves—and the relationships of these selves to split internalized object-images and split external objects. Typical persons with narcissistic personality organization repeatedly behave in such a way as to receive external support for their grandiose selves, which remain inflated while the existence of the hungry selves is denied. Salman Akhtar (1992) has detailed the division of overt and covert aspects of personality that are so persistently displayed in cases like Leo's and Rebecca's. Leo, like Rebecca, endured a traumatic childhood and was thought of by his parents as an exceptional carrier of the Holocaust legacy. His parents' concretized images of Nazis and the Holocaust were deposited in him, "actualizing" those images within his core identity. What made his internal world unusual was his use of images of Nazi omnipotence as a glue to fuse the three elements that comprise and maintain a grandiose self. Nazi power fueled his "specialness," his idealization of aspects of himself and internalized object images; Jewishness formed part of his hungry self. In Rebecca's case, her devalued aspects were overt, while her omnipotently sadistic Nazi aspect was covert but personified; for Leo, the reverse was true. In both cases, however, the grandiose self fused with the image of a Nazi victimizer, while the hungry self fused with the image of a Jewish victim. Though these splits expressed themselves in Leo's and Rebecca's "secret," nonpublic mental worlds, such "private" worlds do on occasion intrude into patients' "public" ones—creating, as we have seen, many interpersonal difficulties.

Leo and Rebecca were different from typical persons with narcissistic personality organizations, insofar as they were *malignant narcissists*, people who need to have what Volkan and Ast (1994) term *aggressive triumphs* in their interpersonal relationships in order to maintain and protect their grandiose selves internally. Leo had to have such triumphs daily in small but steady doses. By aggressively devaluing his therapist or by "banging" women instead of making love to them, for example, he preserved an illusion of supreme power, with no room for shame and humiliation. Before analysis, Leo was doomed to repeat acts of aggressive triumph. Rebecca, on the other hand, could sustain her masochistic aspects for days or months until her sadistic aspect could surface and strike at the cats. Unlike Leo, Rebecca shared certain characteristics with people suffering from *dissociative identity disorder* (DID) (Brenner, 1999b, 2000), who develop "alter personalities"—or, to use Ronald Fairbain's (1952) term, *personifications*. Aspects of herself and her internalized object-images, as happens with patients with DID, were personified as Dr. Mengele and various cats. Ira Brenner (1999b, 2000) describes this phenomenon in another context as the "'It's not me!' self": "an unconscious construct that essentially creates the alters, while tricking the patient into believing that they are not part of her/him, much the way 'the man behind the curtain' wanted to be ignored while he created an illusion of the Wizard of Oz" (Brenner, 1999b, p. 346). Rebecca created the illusion of being a masochist, while behind the curtain she was a sadist.

Rena Moses-Hrushovski (1994) would describe patients such as Leo, Rebecca, and Uta as using *deployment* to console or compensate themselves for what they have experienced in the past as unfair, painful, and humiliating. She argues that deployment entails a rigid self-organization (*not* necessarily an integrated self-organization as we know it) involving a system of attitudes, roles, and behaviors aimed at protecting self-esteem. Individuals who develop this character defense—often in response to overwhelming and humiliating traumas—possess an exaggerated sense of mission to escape disruptive aspects of their internal world. The result is that their perceptions, feelings, and choices are restricted, often leading to self-defeating behavior.

Deployment, then, according to Moses-Hrushovski, is an antithesis of mourning; it reflects unconscious efforts to harden oneself and to deny loss. The individuals' endless vigilance, repeated activities, frozen perspective, sense of righteousness, and use of violence and counter-shame strategies enable them to control emotions associated with guilt, humiliation, uncertainty, sadness, and fear at the expense of empathy, sympathy, and obligation. Pathologically deployed persons behave like soldiers, carrying out the duties they feel are assigned even when these orders run contrary to what the individuals are told by their conscience. Driven to a frenzy of activity, they enact their exhausting programs by becoming "workaholics" or by developing an all-consuming devotion to religion or other ideology. As was shown, Leo's, Rebecca's, and Uta's personally traumatic childhoods led to pathological deployment in adulthood. Their compulsive acts served to maintain both their grandiose selves and their hungry selves, but what is most interesting here is that those acts also actualized images of Jewish and Gypsy victims and Nazi victimizers: Their developmental traumas were condensed with their large groups' respective historical traumas. Martin Bergmann (1982), Anita Eckstaedt (1989), and Ilany Kogan (1995, 2000) provide additional studies of patients who compulsively repeat what has been deposited in them by parents traumatized under the Third Reich.

Treatment of "Difficult" Cases

Analysts and therapists should never adopt the position that deployers, those who are prone to compulsive acts, and those who possess severe narcissistic conditions infused with extreme sadism and masochism cannot be treated. Treatment *is* possible—though in addition to the obstacles mentioned in relation to "mild" cases, which are applicable here as well, the analyst or therapist is required to develop a tolerance for the patient's exaggerated transference expressions and, more difficult, for the analyst's own exaggerated countertransference responses (Boyer, 1983, 1999; Racker, 1968; Searles, 1979). Conventionally, countertransference refers to the analyst's feelings about, perceptions of, and attitudes toward the patient that are actually displacements from the analyst's own early life situations onto the patient. The "totalistic" view of countertransference invoked here, however, includes all of the analyst's feelings, perceptions, and behavior—conscious and unconscious—induced by the patient's transference to the analyst and by whatever actions the patient takes toward the analyst (Boyer, 1983, 1999; Giovacchini, 2000; Kernberg, 1984; Volkan, 1987; Volkan and Ast, 1992, 1994). In order to understand their patients' internal worlds accurately, analysts and therapists must constantly monitor their own reactions to patients' behavior, including, as was discussed, any effects of the therapist's own large-group identity.

Indeed, as shown in the case studies, more difficult patients tend to communicate the influence of Holocaust and Nazi images primarily through actions, rather than words. The transference relationship thus frequently becomes a stage on which the ancestors' drama is enacted, and, for a time, the patient "forces" the therapist or analyst to participate as an actor in this drama. When therapists or analysts find themselves under some internal pressure to depart from standard psychoanalytic technique in order to accommodate patients, however, these clinicians must thoroughly understand the active countertransference at work. At one point during Leo's treatment, for example, Dr. Greer discovered that he had fallen under the "spell" of Leo's internal world. Even though Dr. Greer knew the correct technical response to Leo's imperious demands for answers to questions, he found himself feeling temporarily powerless in the face of Leo's efforts to control him. Indeed, the analyst found himself obsessively rehearsing each potential interaction; in a sense, like Leo, he had lost his capacity to verbalize and think through his experiences. In both his mind and his patient's, he had become identified with the helpless, frightened Jewish victim, while Leo had become identified with the omnipotent Nazi persecutor whose murderous rage the analyst dared not arouse. Until Dr. Greer could symbolize the protosymbolic nature of his interactions with Leo, his apprehension permeated the therapeutic relationship, hindering the patient's progress. Once Dr. Greer understood, through self-analysis, his reaction to Leo's behavior, he dis-identified himself from the Jewish victim-image and was able to recover his analytic functions.

Anita Eckstaedt (1989) reports a more painful and potentially difficult example of countertransference response in the course of treating a Third Reich–related case: fear induced by feeling forced to see herself as a potential murderer. But it is only through "tolerance"—in other words, only through the therapeutic management of such exaggerated transference and countertransference manifestations—that the analytic position can be maintained. The analyst or psychotherapist who tolerates countertransference feelings and refrains from involvement in the many crises the patient brings to treatment can keep the therapeutic space safe from intrusions. Uta's and Leo's cases provide examples of analysts effectively protecting and maintaining the therapeutic position and space (though doing so was simply not possible when the reality of Dr. Greer's cancer impinged on Leo's case; how Dr. Greer recreated the appropriate analytic space is described in chapter 6). Leo's prior analyst provides a counter-example resulting in adverse outcomes. Obviously, one cannot command therapists or analysts to be tolerant when malignant narcissists sadistically attack them repeatedly during each session; the analysts' or the therapists' proper training sustains them in these situations. Because of the intense pressure that these patients can create in analysts and therapists, however, we do strongly advise proper supervision for those therapists inexperienced in handling complex patterns of transference and countertransference.

Whatever advanced ego functions "difficult" patients may exhibit—for example, both Uta and Leo were quite competent in their respective workplaces, and Leo is a highly intellectual person indeed—their reality-testing is blurred at a certain level. When people who live in both the present and the past plunge into a life in the "secret," past world, they construe self- and object-images not as symbols that stand for those images, but as felt equivalents to them; the internal referent and the external object are undifferentiated. In such individuals, thought has not achieved its more developed status as trial-action; they concretize mental content in action and are therefore unable to examine it with any affective distance. Because, in the cases described here, one of the worlds belongs to the ancestor's lifetime and is no longer real, the patient who lives in it needs to make that world exist only as a mental representation in memory—that is, as a world expressed in symbols. Interpreting why a patient has developed a sadistic grandiose self and masochistic hungry self or why a patient constantly uses deployment—while also necessary when the patient is ready to "hear" it—is simply not enough to cure such patients. Because the patients utilize Third Reich– or Holocaust-related images as pure protosymbols or as protosymbols with some symbolic functions, the transference that contains such images is not a typical workable transference neurosis or even a narcissistic transference workable by means of interpretations only. Mental content that has become concretized in action must be transformed into abstract symbolic thought for the transference to become more workable. The patient and the analyst, as protosymbols of Nazi images in the patient's internal world, need to "play" together in the therapeutic space, with the analyst regressing "in the service of the other" (Olinick, 1969), while remaining the protector of that space (see also Giovacchini, 2000; Volkan and Ast, 1994).

Albert Solnit (1987) has suggested that "play" is "better described by its functions" (p. 205) than by theoretical formulation. As might be expected, the psychoanalytic literature includes more exploration of the function of play among children and technical implications of playing in child analysis (Marans, Mayes, and Colonna, 1993, provide a comprehensive summary of psychoanalytic views of children's play) than of its functions for adults and technical implications for adult analysis. Wondering how understanding the role of play in child analysis might relate to analytic treatment for adults, Peter Neubauer (1993) suggests that if we consider play "to be an attempt at a solution of conflicts, of the establishment of ego mastery, whether this is done in action, words, or fantasy, then we find a more common ground that links child and adult analysis" (p. 51). Through action or daydream, an adult patient's "therapeutic play" evolves a story from session to session that helps the patient assimilate insight, evolve protosymbols into symbols, develop the ability to tame and tolerate aggression, increase the capacity for mourning, and learn to master reality (Volkan and Ast, in press). In the process, a transference neurosis (at times, a transference psychosis) develops, in which the patient's unreal world "comes to life" within the sessions with appropriate affects, including countertransference affects that need to be employed therapeutically rather than as tools for the analyst's or therapist's own acting-out. Thus the therapist properly becomes in therapeutic play a "transitional object" (Winnicott, 1953), "a temporary construction to aid [the patient] in the early stages of developing a sense of reality and establishing his own individual identity" (Greenacre, 1970, p. 334). Patients with "concretized" (Bergmann, 1982; Kogan, 1995, 2000) unconscious fantasies pertaining to the Third Reich need to re-experience their childhood traumas rather tangibly within the transference and work through them so that they can stop expecting the return of their traumas with Nazi-related protosymbols. Uta and Dr. Ast's 4-month play with the patient's "ghost" provides a fine example (see chapter 7). Once the "play" ends, the patient develops a capacity for mourning and ability to test reality; now the analyst's interpretations can be effective.

When developing interpretations, it is important for the analyst to recall that the primary conflicts of those, like Leo, who have malignant narcissistic personality organization are preoedipal. Initially, then, such patients exhibit more object-relations conflict than structural (id-ego-superego) conflicts and suffer more from separation anxiety than castration anxiety. As analysts follow the technical axiom of going from surface to depth, they need to keep in mind that what is on the surface for such patients are developmentally primitive phenomena. Such patients' splitting, denial, projective identification, and omnipotent control mechanisms will therefore require the therapist's or analyst's initial attention—*before* repression and related high-level defense mechanisms such as intellectualization, rationalization, and isolation.

Eventually, though, such patients begin to have crucial juncture experiences. Borrowed from the work of Melanie Klein (1946), the term *crucial juncture* designates a moment in analysis in which unintegrated (borderline or narcissistic) patients attempt to integrate their opposing self- and object-images and associated opposing affect derivatives. Another of Dr. Volkan's patients (1991b; see also Volkan and Ast, 1992) metaphorized the crucial juncture experience as that of a Mafia man fed lavishly, kissed on the lips, and then summarily killed; one minute the man was loved, and the next minute he was destroyed. For this patient, who had extensively used splitting mechanisms, the notion of "love" and "hate" meeting at one point was a new idea. In Uta's and Leo's cases, opposing self- and object-images and associated opposing affect derivatives were expressed through Jenish/Jewish/victim and Nazi/victimizer images. Leo, for instance, attempted to bring such opposing images and associated affect together in a dream about and temporary identification with the actor Christopher Reeve. For this patient, to refer to the accident in which Reeve, who had played Superman in the movies (powerful Aryan/Nazi), had been paralyzed (Jewish victim) was to identify a point at which "omnipotence" and "victimhood" could meet.

In order to reach the crucial juncture, it is necessary for the patient to identify with the analyst's reality-testing, integrating, abstracting, and taming ego-functions. Patients are likely to resist such identifications, since they continue to contaminate their analysts with their own externalized images and projected thoughts, perceptions, and affects. These patients will have trouble differentiating their analysts' roles as transference figures from the analysts' roles as "new objects" (Kernberg, 1975; Leowald, 1960; Volkan, 1976). But patients can eventually perceive the "newness" of the analyst—that is, can, through their interactions with the analyst or therapist, "rediscover . . . the early paths of the development of object-relations leading to a new way of relating to objects and of being oneself" (Leowald, 1960, p. 20). It is necessary for such patients to undergo multiple crucial juncture experiences in order to achieve integrated self- and object-representations and to develop a healthy narcissism—the ability to maintain self-esteem without inflating the grandiose self or externalizing the humiliated hungry self (or even vice versa). They can now accept their own true "averageness," especially their aggression's ordinariness. Once this integration is achieved, the patient can then be treated like any person with a neurotic personality organization, and interpretation becomes the primary tool in the analysis, as occurred in both Uta's and Leo's cases. Rebecca also needed to integrate her self-concept, but we do not know whether she would be able do so, since she has refused to undergo psychoanalytic treatment.

After experiencing enough crucial junctures, "difficult patients" are, then, on the path to further improvement when they experience, in the workable transference neurosis, separation-individuation struggles (Mahler, 1968) for the first time with their newly "integrated" self-representations (that is, assimilation of previously unintegrated self- and object-images to their already-integrated aspects of core identity) and a healthy narcissism. At the same time, analysts or psychotherapists will observe that patients are beginning to give up their reenactments and starting to put the influence of traumatic experiences into words—that is, experiencing a shift from protosymbolic to symbolic mentation. Only at this point does the patient truly have a mind that can contain, reflect upon, and verbalize its own contents. Finally, the patient experiences oedipal conflicts and resolutions (as was seen in Uta's case, especially), again for the first time with healthy narcissism and cohesive identity; such processes themselves further crystallize cohesive identity. Moreover, patients develop further capacity to mourn as "normal" adults, and, when the termination phase is reached, they are able to let the analysts go. The newly increased capacity for mourning is also reflected in the way the patients confront their "loss" of the actualized influences of Third Reich or Holocaust images buried in their identities. The "memories" of these images are not forgotten; they are forever part of the patient's personal and large-group identity. But they do cease to exercise their commanding grip on the patient's mental life.

Afterword
RAMIFICATIONS

DURING THE SUMMERS OF 1998 AND 1999, Dr. Volkan participated in a series of small-group meetings in Dubrovnik, Croatia, among Croatian, Serbian, and Bosniak psychiatrists and psychologists organized by Professor Eduard Klain of the University of Zagreb. The gatherings were designed to help local mental health professionals become better caretakers by exploring their own ethnic attitudes and traumas in a process similar to the one that Dr. Volkan formulated for the PAKH core group meetings discussed in chapter 9 of this book. Since traumas in the former Yugoslavia were fresh, the Croatian, Serbian, and Bosniak colleagues came to the meetings holding firmly to their respective large-group identities, acting as spokespersons for their ethnic groups. Needless to say, these meetings were very intense.

Dr. Klain had also invited a group of Israeli psychoanalysts and other mental health professionals, including Shalom Litman, Dina Wardi, and Judith Stern, to take part in these meetings. After much discussion of the traumatized Croatian, Serbian, and Bosniak patients that these indigenous caretakers were treating, and after examining the caretakers' own traumas, the Israelis powerfully warned those present of another major issue: the transgenerational transmission of trauma. The Israelis reminded their Croatian, Serbian, and Bosniak colleagues that it had taken the Israeli mental health community two or three decades after the end of World War II to work through their own denials sufficiently to understand that the second and third generations after the Holocaust needed close attention and care as well. "Let us give you some advice," admonished the Israelis. "You don't need to wait 10 or 20 years to develop strategies to deal with the next generation."

What the Israeli mental health workers told their colleagues from the former Yugoslavia needs to be taken very seriously. Much as we may hope for the end of large-group historical traumas, recent events in the Balkans, the Caucasus, Rwanda, Burundi, Indonesia, Chechnya, and elsewhere indicate that we are far from seeing the last of shared immiseration. Though the atrocities of the Nazi regime are historically unique in their nature and magnitude, we emphatically affirm that the study of how transgenerational transmissions have occurred in their aftermath can be useful in developing strategies (Volkan, 1999e) to prevent maladaptive and even malignant transmissions at the large-group level after any massive ethnic or national trauma and evolution of chosen trauma. The necessary strategies will likely require mental health professionals to work in interdisciplinary teams that include historians, political scientists, diplomats, social scientists, and others. Such experiments have been ongoing at the University of Virginia School of Medicine's Center for the Study of Mind and Human Interaction (CSMHI) for the past 12 years. We hope that this book, which focuses on the individual's mental life, can provide a useful stepping-stone in the processes of crafting those strategies, not only by illustrating important aspects of the intertwined relationship of individual psychology and large-group psychology, but also by stimulating further thought on the precise forms of "preventive medicine" (Volkan, 1999e, 2000) that mental health professionals may be able to administer—and for which diplomats, political scientists, and others may advocate—following future massive war or warlike traumas, in order to avert maladaptive societal responses that reverberate across the decades and centuries to come. If psychoanalysts are unable to prevent the traumas of the fathers and mothers from being visited upon the children, as Exodus 20:5 has it, "unto the third and fourth generation," our profession may well be able, at least, to tame the malignant influences of their transgenerational transmissions.

References

Abraham, K. (1949). *Selected papers on psychoanalysis*, ed. D. Bryan & A. Strachey. London: Hogarth Press.

Abraham, M. (1988). Notes on the phantom. In F. Meltzer (Ed.), *The trials of psychoanalysis* (pp. 75–80). Chicago: Chicago University Press.

Abse, D. W. (1974). *Clinical notes on group-analytic psychotherapy*. Charlottesville: University Press of Virginia.

Ainsworth, M., Bell, S. M., & Stayton, D. (1974). Infant–mother attachment and social development: Socialization as a product of reciprocal responsiveness to signals. In M. Richards (Ed.), *The integration of the child into a social world* (pp. 99–135). Cambridge, England: Cambridge University Press.

Akhtar, S. (1992). *Broken structures: Severe personality disorders and their treatment*. Northvale, NJ: Jason Aronson.

Akhtar, S. (1995). The third individuation, immigration, identity and psychoanalytic process. *Journal of the American Psychoanalytic Association*, *43*, 1051–1084.

Akhtar, S. (1999). *Immigration and identity*. Northvale, NJ: Jason Aronson.

Akhtar, S., & Samuel, S. (1996). The concept of identity: Developmental origins, phenomenology, clinical relevance and measurement. *Harvard Review of Psychiatry*, *3*, 254–267.

Apprey, M. (1993a). The African-American experience: Forced immigration and transgenerational trauma. *Mind and Human Interaction*, *4*, 70–75.

Apprey, M. (1993b). Dreams of urgent-voluntary errands and transgenerational haunting and transsexualism. In M. Apprey & H. F. Stein (Eds.), *Intersubjectivity, projective identification, and otherness* (pp. 102–128). Pittsburgh, PA: Duquesne University Press.

Apprey, M. (1996). Heuristic steps for negotiating ethno-national conflicts: Vignettes from Estonia. *New Literary History*, *27*, 199–212.

Apprey, M., Krikk, L., Apprey, V., & Talvik, E. (2000). From the heuristic to the empirical: Integrating interethnic kindergartens. *Mind and Human Interaction*, *11*, 195–207.

Appy, J-G. (1993). The meaning of "Auschwitz" today: Clinical reflections about the depletion of a destructive symbol. In R. Moses (Ed.), *Persistent shadows of the Holocaust: The meaning to those not directly affected* (pp. 3–36). Madison, CT: International University Press.

Arlow, J. (1969). Unconscious fantasy and disturbances of conscious experience. *Psychoanalytic Quarterly, 38,* 1–27.

Ash, T. G. (1998). Diktatur und Wahrheit: Die Suche nach Gerechtigkeit und die Politik der Erinnerung (Dictatorship and truth: Looking for justice and the politics of remembering). *Lettre International, 10,* 10–15.

Ast, G. (1991). Interviews with Germans about reunification. *Mind and Human Interaction, 2,* 100–104.

Auerhahn, N. C., & Laub, D. (1998). The primal scene of atrocity: The dynamic interplay between knowledge and fantasy of the Holocaust in children of survivors. *Psychoanalytic Psychology, 15,* 360–377.

Bar-On, D. (1989). *Legacy of silence: Encounters with children of the Third Reich.* Cambridge, MA: Harvard University Press.

Beres, D. (1962). The unconscious fantasy. *Psychoanalytic Quarterly, 31,* 309–329.

Bergmann, M. S. (1982). Thoughts on super-ego pathology of survivors and their children. In M. S. Bergmann & M. E. Jucovy (Eds.), *Generations of the Holocaust* (pp. 287–311). New York: Basic Books.

Bernard, W. W., Ottenberg, P., & Redl, F. (1973). Dehumanization: A composite psychological defense in relation to modern war. In N. Sanford & C. Comstock (Eds.), *Sanctions for evil: Sources of social destructiveness* (pp. 102–124). San Francisco: Jossey-Bass.

Bettelheim, B. (1960). *The informed heart.* Glencoe, IL: Free Press of Glencoe.

Bion, W. R. (1961). *Experiences in groups.* London: Tavistock Publications.

Blos, P. (1979). *The adolescent passage.* New York: International Universities Press.

Blum, H. P. (1985). Superego formation, adolescent transformation and the adult neurosis. *Journal of the American Psychoanalytic Association, 4,* 887–909

Bocksel, A. A. (1991). *Rice, men and barbed wire: A true epic of Americans as Japanese POW's.* Hauppage, NY: Michael B. Glass & Associates.

Bowlby, J. (1960). Grief and mourning in infancy and early childhood. *The Psychoanalytic Study of the Child, 15,* 9–52. New York: International Universities Press.

Bowlby, J. (1969). *Attachment and loss.* Vol. 1: *Attachment.* New York: Basic Books.

Boyer, C. B. (1983). *The regressed patient.* New York: Jason Aronson.

Boyer, C. B. (1999). *Countertransference and regression.* Northvale, NJ: Jason Aronson.

Brazelton, T., Koslowski, B., & Main, N. (1974). The origins of reciprocity: The early mother–infant interaction. In M. Lewis & L. Rosenblum (Eds.), *The effects of the infant on its caregiver* (pp. 49–76). New York: John Wiley.

Breloer, H. (1997). *Todesspiel: Von der Schleyer-Entführung bis Mogadischu: Eine dokumentarische Erzählung* (Death game: From the kidnapping of Schleyer to Mogadischu: A documentary re-creation). Köln: Verlag Kiepenheuer & Witsch.

Brenner, I. (1988). Unconscious fantasies of the selection in children of Holocaust survivors. Paper presented at the First International Conference of Children of Holocaust Survivors, Jerusalem. December.

Brenner, I. (1991). On confronting the truth about the Third Reich. *Mind and Human Interaction, 2,* 97–100.

Brenner, I. (1999a). Returning to the fire: Surviving the Holocaust and "going back." *Journal of Applied Psychoanalytic Studies, 1,* 145–162.

Brenner, I. (1999b). Deconstructing DID. *American Journal of Psychotherapy, 53,* 344–360.

Brenner, I. (2000). *Incest, injury, insight and integration: Studies in dissociated trauma.* Madison, CT: International Universities Press.

Brown, E. M. (1998). The transmission of trauma through caretaking patterns of behavior in Holocaust families: Re-enactments in a facilitated long-term second-generation group. *Smith College Studies in Social Work, 68,* 267–285.

Cain, A. C., & Cain, B. S. (1964). On replacing a child. *Journal of the American Academy of Child Psychiatry, 3,* 443–456.

Chodoff, P. (1963). Late effects of the concentration camp syndrome. *Archives of General Psychiatry, 8,* 323–333.

Chodoff, P. (1970). The German concentration camp as a psychological stress. *Archives of General Psychiatry, 22,* 78–87.

Danieli, Y. (1989). Mourning in survivors and children of survivors of the Nazi Holocaust: The role of group and community modalities. In D. R. Dietrich & P. C. Shabad (Eds.), *The problem of loss and mourning* (pp. 427–460). Madison, CT: International Universities Press.

Deri, S. (1978). Transitional phenomenon: Vicissitudes of symbolization and creativity. In S. A. Grolnick & L. Barkin (Eds.), *Between reality and fantasy* (pp. 43–80). New York: Jason Aronson.

de Wind, E. (1968). The confrontation with death. *International Journal of Psycho-Analysis, 49,* 302–305.

Eckstaedt, A. (1989). *Nationalsozialismus in der "zweiten Generation": Psychoanalyse von Hörigkeitsverhältnissen* (National socialism in the second generation: Psychoanalysis of master–slave relationships). Frankfurt a.M.: Suhrkamp Verlag.

Eiber, L. (1993). *Ich wusste, es wird schlimm* (I knew it would become awful). München: Buchendorfer Verlag.

Eissler, K. R. (1963). Die Ermordung von wievielen seiner Kinder muß ein Mensch symptomfrei ertragen können, um eine normale Konstitution zu haben? (The murder of how many of his own children does a person have to be able to tolerate without developing symptoms in order to have a normal constitution?) *Psyche, 17,* 241–291.

Eitinger, L. (1961). Pathology of the concentration camp syndrome. *Archives of General Psychiatry, 5,* 371–379.

Eitinger, L. (1964). *Concentration camp survivors in Norway and Israel.* London: Allen & Unwin.

Emde, R. N. (1988a). Development terminable and interminable. 1. Innate and motivational factors from infancy. *International Journal of Psycho-Analysis, 69,* 23–41.

Emde, R. N. (1988b). Development terminable and interminable. 2. Recent psychoanalytic theory and therapeutic considerations. *International Journal of Psycho-Analysis, 69,* 283–296.

Emde, R. N. (1991). Positive emotions for psychoanalytic theory: Surprises from infancy research and new directions. *Journal of the American Psychoanalytic Association* (Supplement), *39,* 5–44.

Emmert, T. A. (1990). *Serbian Golgotha: Kosovo, 1389.* New York: Columbia University Press.

Erikson, E. H. (1954). The dream specimen of psychoanalysis. In R. P. Knight & C. R. Friedman (Eds.), *Psychoanalytic psychiatry and psychology: Austen Riggs Center, Vol. 1* (pp. 131–170). New York: International Universities Press.

Erikson, E. H. (1956). The problem of ego identification. *Journal of the American Psychoanalytic Association, 4*, 56–121.

Erikson, K. T. (1975). Loss of communality at Buffalo Creek. *American Journal of Psychiatry, 133*, 302–325.

Fairbain, W. R. D. (1952). *Psychoanalytic studies of the personality*. Boston: Routledge and Kegan Paul.

Fenichel, O. (1945). *The psychoanalytic theory of neurosis*. New York: Norton.

Fings, K., Heuss, H., & Sparing, F. (1997). *From "race science" to the camps: The gypsies during the Second World War* (D. Kenrick, Trans.). Hertfordshire, England: University of Hertfordshire Press.

Fink, F. H. (1968). Developmental arrest as a result of Nazi persecution during adolescence. *International Journal of Psycho-Analysis, 49*, 327–329.

Foulkes, S. H., & Anthony, E. J. (1957). *Group psychotherapy*. London: Penguin Books.

Freud, A. (1960). Discussion of Dr. John Bowlby's paper. *The Psychoanalytic Study of the Child, 15*, 53–62. New York: International Universities Press.

Freud, A. & Burlingham, D. (1942). *War and children*. New York: International Universities Press.

Freud, S. (1887–1902). *The origins of psychoanalysis: Letters to Wilhelm Fliess, drafts and notes: 1887–1902* (M. Bonaparte, A. Freud, & E. Kris, Eds.). New York: Basic Books, 1954.

Freud, S. (1908). Hysterical phantasies and their relation to bisexuality. *Standard Edition, 9*, 155–166. London: Hogarth Press, 1959.

Freud, S. (1917a). Taboo of virginity. *Standard Edition, 11*, 191–208. London: Hogarth Press, 1961.

Freud, S. (1917b). Mourning and melancholia. *Standard Edition, 14*, 237–258. London: Hogarth Press, 1961.

Freud, S. (1921). Group psychology and the analysis of the ego. *Standard Edition, 18*, 16–143. London: Hogarth Press, 1955.

Freud, S. (1923). The ego and the id. *Standard Edition, 19*, 3–66. London: Hogarth Press, 1961.

Freud, S. (1925). An autobiographical study. *Standard Edition*, 20, 7–74. London: Hogarth Press, 1959.

Freud, S. (1926). Inhibitions, symptoms and anxiety. *Standard Edition*, 20, 77–175. London: Hogarth Press, 1959.

Freud, S. (1927). Fetishism. *Standard Edition, 21*, 149–157. London: Hogarth Press, 1964.

Freud, S. (1930). Civilization and its discontents. *Standard Edition 21*, 59–145. London: Hogarth Press, 1964.

Freud, S. (1940). Splitting of the ego in the process of defence. *Standard Edition, 23*, 271–278. London: Hogarth Press, 1964.

Friedman, P. (1949). Some aspects of concentration camp psychology. *American Journal of Psychiatry, 105*, 601–605.

Giovacchini, P. L. (2000). *Impact of narcissism: The errant therapist on a chaotic quest*. Northvale, NJ: Jason Aronson.

Glover, E. (1955). *Technique of psychoanalysis*. New York: International University Press.

Goenjian, A. K., Steinberg, A. M., Najarian, L. M., Fairbanks, L. A., Tashjian, M., & Pynoos, R. S. (2000). Prospective study of posttraumatic stress, anxiety, and depressive reactions after earthquake and political violence. *American Journal of Psychiatry, 157,* 911–916.

Green, N., & Solnit, A. J. (1964). Reactions to the threatened loss of a child: A vulnerable child syndrome. *Pediatrics, 34,* 58–66.

Greenacre, P. (1970). The transitional object and the fetish: With special reference to the role of illusion. *International Journal of Psycho-Analysis, 51,* 447–456.

Greenspan, S. I. (1989). *The development of the ego: Implications for personality theory, psychopathology and the psychotherapeutic process.* Madison, CT: International Universities Press.

Grinberg, L., & Grinberg, R. (1989). *Psychoanalytic perspectives on migration and exile* (N. Festinger, Trans.). New Haven, CT: Yale University Press.

Gross, H. (1899). Das Gaunerglossar der Freistädter Handscrift (The glossary of scoundrels of the Freistädter manuscript). In *Archiv für Kriminal-Anthropologie und Kriminalistik, Band 2* (Vol. 2). Leipzig: Verlag Vogel.

Grubrich-Simitis, I. (1979). Extremtraumatisierung als kumulatives Trauma. Psychoanalytische Studien über seelische Nachwirkungen der Konzentrationslagerhaft bei Überlebenden und ihren Kindern (Extreme traumatization as a cumulative trauma. Psychoanalytic studies of the mental effects of imprisonment in concentration camps on survivors and their children). *Psyche, 33,* 991–1023.

Hartmann, H. (1950). Comments on the psychoanalytic theory of the ego. In *Essays on Ego Psychology* (pp. 113–141). New York: International Universities Press, 1964.

Heath, S. (1991). *Dealing with the therapist's vulnerability to depression.* Northvale, NJ: Jason Aronson.

Hitler, A. (1930). *Mein Kampf, Band 1 und 2* (My struggle, Vols. 1 and 2). München: F. Eher Nachf. Verlag.

Hoppe, K. D. (1966). The psychodynamics of concentration camp victims. *Psychoanalytic Forum, 1,* 75–80.

Hoppe, K. D. (1968). Re-somatization of affects in survivors of persecution. *International Journal of Psycho-Analysis, 49,* 324–326.

Horowitz, M. J. (1986). *Stress response syndrome.* Northvale, NJ: Jason Aronson.

Inderbitzin, L. B., & Levy, S. T. (1990). Unconscious fantasy: A reconsideration of the concept. *Journal of the American Psychoanalytic Association, 38,* 113–130.

Jacobson, E. (1964). *The self and the object world.* New York: International Universities Press.

Jaffe, R. (1968). Dissociative phenomena in former concentration camp inmates. *International Journal of Psycho-Analysis, 49,* 310–312.

Jokl, A. M. (1997). *Zwei Fälle zum Thema "Bewältigung der Vergangenheit"* (Two cases referring to the theme of "mastering the past"). Frankfurt a. M.: Jüdischer Verlag.

Jucovy, M. (1998). The background of persecution and its aftermath. In J. S. Kestenberg & C. Kahn (Eds.), *Children surviving persecution: An international study of trauma and healing* (pp. 19–42). Westport, CT: Praeger.

Jütte, R. (1988). *Abbild und soziale Wirklichkeit des Bettler- und Gaunertums zu Beginn der Neuzeit: Sozial-, mentalitäts- und sprachgeschichtliche Studien zum Liber Vagatorum (1510)* (The image and social reality of beggars and petty criminals at the beginning of the modern age: Social, mentality and linguistic studies referring to Liber Vagatorum [1510]). Köln: Böhlau Verlag.

Kenrick, D., & Puxon, G. (1995). *Gypsies under the swastika*. Hertfordshire, England: University of Hertfordshire Press.

Kernberg, O. F. (1970). Factors in the psychoanalytic treatment of narcissistic personalities. *Journal of the American Psychoanalytic Association, 18*, 51–85.

Kernberg, O. F. (1975). *Borderline conditions and pathological narcissism*. New York: Jason Aronson.

Kernberg, O. F. (1980). *Internal world and external reality*. New York: Jason Aronson.

Kernberg, O. F. (1984). *Severe personality disorders: Psychotherapeutic strategies*. New Haven: Yale University Press.

Kestenberg, J. S. (1982). A psychological assessment based on analysis of a survivor's child. In M. S. Bergmann & M. E. Jucovy (Eds.), *Generations of the Holocaust* (pp. 177–158). New York: Columbia University Press.

Kestenberg, J. S. (1989). Coping with losses and survival. In D. R. Dietrich & P. C. Shabad (Eds.), *The problem of loss and mourning: Psychoanalytic perspectives* (pp. 381–403). Madison, CT: International Universities Press.

Kestenberg, J., & Brenner, I. (1996). *The last witness*. Washington, DC: American Psychiatric Press.

Klein, M. (1946). Notes on some schizoid mechanisms. *International Journal of Psycho-Analysis, 27*, 99–110.

Kogan, I. (1995). *The cry of mute children: A psychoanalytic perspective of the second generation of the Holocaust*. London: Free Association Books.

Kogan, I. (2000). Breaking the cycle of trauma—From the individual to society. *Mind and Human Interaction, 11*, 2–10.

Krystal, H. (Ed.). (1968). *Massive psychic trauma*. New York: International Universities Press.

Kuhn, A., Staemmler, M., & Burgdorfer, F. (1938). *Erbkunde, Rassenpflege, Bevölkerungspolitik: Schicksalsfragen des deutschen Volkes* (Genetics, care and attention of the race, population politics: Fateful questions of/for the German people). Leipzig: Verlag Quelle & Meyer.

Lazarovich-Hrebelianovich, P., & Calhoun, E. (1910). *The Serbian people*. Vol. 1. New York: Scribner's.

Legg, L. A., & Sherick, I. (1976). The replacement child—A developmental tragedy: Some preliminary comments. *Child Psychiatry and Human Development, 7*, 79–97.

Lehtonen, J. (1999). Personal communications with Dr. Volkan.

Lehtonen, J., Könönen, M., Purhonen, M., Partanen, J., Saarikoski, S., & Launiala, K. (1998). The effect of nursing on the brain activity of the newborn. *Journal of Pediatrics, 132*, 646–651.

Leowald, H. (1960). On the therapeutic action of psychoanalysis. *International Journal of Psycho-Analysis, 41*, 16–33.

Liégeois, J-P. (1994). *Roma, gypsies, travellers*. Strasbourg: Council of Europe Press.

Lifton, R. J. (1968). *Death in life: Survivors of Hiroshima*. New York: Random House.

Lifton, R.J., & Olson, E. (1976). The human meaning of total disaster: The Buffalo Creek experience. *Psychiatry, 39*, 1–18.

Lorenzer, A. (1968). Some observations on the latency of symptoms in patients suffering from persecution sequelae. *International Journal of Psycho-Analysis, 49*, 316–318.

Lübbe, H. (1983). Der Nationalsozialismus im deutschen Nachkriegsbewußtein (National Socialism in the German postwar consciousness). *Historische Zeitschrift, 236,* 579–599.

Mahler, M. S. (1968). *On human symbiosis and the vicissitudes of individuation.* New York: International Universities Press.

Marans, S., Mayes, L. C., & Colonna, A. B. (1993). Psychoanalytic views of children's play. In A. J. Solnit, D. J. Cohen, & P. B. Neubauer (Eds.), *The many meanings of play: A psychoanalytic perspective* (pp. 9–28). New Haven: Yale University Press.

Margalit, G. (1997). Postscript. In K. Fings, H. Heuss, & F. Sparing, *From "race science" to the camps: The gypsies during the Second World War* (D. Kenrick, Trans.) (pp. 110–111). Hertfordshire, England: University of Hertfordshire Press.

Markovic, M. S. (1983). The secret of Kosovo. In V. D. Mihailovich (Ed.), *Landmarks in Serbian culture and history* (C. Kramer, Trans.) (pp. 111–131). Pittsburgh, PA: Serb National Federation.

Meyer, E. (1990). A "nest-befouler," *Jerusalem Post International Edition,* December 1.

Mitscherlich, A., & Mitscherlich, M. (1975). *The inability to mourn: Principals of collective behavior* (B. R. Placzek, Trans.). New York: Grove Press, 1967.

Mitscherlich-Nielsen, M. (1979). Die Notwendigkeit zu trauern (The necessity to mourn). *Psyche, 33,* 981–990.

Moore, B. E., & Fine, B. D. (1990). *Psychoanalytic terms and concepts.* New Haven, CT: Yale University Press.

Moser, T. (1992). Die Unfähigkeit zu trauern: Hält die Diagnose einer Überprüfung stand? Zur psychischen Verarbeitung des Holocausts in der Bundesrepublik (The inability to mourn: Does the diagnosis withstand scrutiny?). *Psyche, 46,* 389–405.

Moses, R. (1984). An Israeli psychologist looks back in 1983. In S. A. Luel & P. Marcus (Eds.), *Psychoanalytic reflections on the Holocaust: Selected essays* (pp. 52–70). New York: Ktav Publishing House.

Moses, R. (Ed.). (1993). *Persistent shadows of the Holocaust: The meaning to those not directly affected.* Madison, CT: International Universities Press.

Moses, R., & Cohen, Y. (1993). An Israeli view. In R. Moses (Ed.), *Persistent shadows of the Holocaust: The meaning to those not directly affected* (pp. 199–153). Madison, CT: International Universities Press.

Moses-Hrushovski, R. (1994). *Deployment: Hiding behind power struggles as a character defense.* Northvale, NJ: Jason Aronson.

Neu, J., & Volkan, V. D. (1999). *Developing a methodology for conflict prevention: The case of Estonia.* Atlanta: The Carter Center.

Neubauer, P. B. (1993). Playing: Technical implications. In A. J. Solnit, D. J. Cohen, & P. B. Neubauer (Eds.), *The many meanings of play: A psychoanalytic perspective* (pp. 44–53). New Haven: Yale University Press.

Niederland, W. C. (1961). The problem of the survivor. *Journal of the Hillside Hospital, 10,* 233–247.

Niederland, W. C. (1964). Psychiatric disorders among persecution victims. *Journal of Nervous and Mental Disorders, 139,* 458–474.

Niederland, W. C. (1968). Clinical observations on the "survivor syndrome." *International Journal of Psycho-Analysis, 49,* 313–315.

Novey, S. (1968). *The second look: The reconstruction of personal history in psychiatry and psychoanalysis.* Baltimore: Johns Hopkins Press.

Ohlmeier, D. (1990). Unconscious derivatives of the Nazi language in the children of the Nazi generation. Paper presented to Bar Ilan University, School of Social Work, The National Conference on the Holocaust, Israel, May 22–23.

Ohlmeier, D. (1991). The return of the repressed: Psychoanalytical reflections on the unification of Germany. Paper presented to the Sandor Ferenczi Society, Budapest, June 7.

Olinick, S. (1964). The negative therapeutic reaction. *International Journal of Psycho-Analysis, 45,* 540–548.

Olinick, S. (1969). On empathy and regression in the service of the other. *British Journal of Medical Psychology, 42,* 41–49.

Opher-Cohn, L., Pfäfflin, J., Sonntag, B., Klose, B., & Pogany-Wnendt, P. (Eds.) (2000). *Auswirkungen traumatischer Holocaust-Erfahrungen über mehrere Generationen* (The effects of experiencing the Holocaust over several generations). Gießen, Germany: Psychosozial-Verlag.

Ornstein, A. (1985). Survival and recovery. *Psychoanalytic Inquiry, 5,* 99–130.

Pao, P.-N. (1979). *Schizophrenic disorders: Theory and treatment from a psychodynamic point of view.* New York: International Universities Press.

Parens, H. (1999). Some influences of the Holocaust on development—One man's experience. Presented at the Thirtieth Annual Scientific Meeting of the American College of Psychoanalysts, Washington, DC, May 15.

Poland, W. S. (1977). Pilgrimage: Action and tradition in self-analysis. *Journal of the American Psychoanalytic Association, 25,* 319–416.

Pollock, G. H. (1989). *The mourning-liberation process,* Vols. 1 & 2. Madison, CT: International Universities Press.

Pott, A. F. (1844 & 1845). *Die Zigeuner in Europa und Asien* (The Gypsy in Europe and Asia). (Vols. 1 and 2). Halle: Heynemann Verlag.

Poznanski, E. O. (1972). The "replacement child": A saga of unresolved parental grief. *Behavioral Pediatrics, 81,* 1190–1193.

Racker, H. (1968). *Transference and countertransference.* New York: International Universities Press.

Ramati, A. (1986). *And the violins stopped playing: A story of the Gypsy Holocaust.* New York: Franklin Watts.

Rangell, L. (1976). Discussion of Buffalo Creek disaster: The course of psychic trauma. *American Journal of Psychiatry, 133,* 313–316.

Rappaport, E. P. (1968). Beyond traumatic neurosis. *International Journal of Psycho-Analysis, 49,* 719–731.

Ritter, R. (1937). *Ein Menschenschlag: Erbärztliche und erbgeschichtliche Untersuchungen über die durch 10 Geschlechterfolgen erforschten Nachkommen von "Vagabunden, Gaunern, und Räubern"* (A breed: Medical-hereditary and historical-hereditary investigation through 10 generations of descendants of "vagabonds and brigands"). Leipzig: Georg Thime Verlag.

Ritter, R. (1938). Zigeuner und Landfahrer (Gypsies and Travelers). In *Der nicht se ßhafte Mensch* (Those who are not sedentary). München: Beck.

Ritter, R. (1939). Die Zigeunerfrage und das Zigeunerbastardproblem (The Gypsy question and the problem of Gypsy bastards). In *Rassenhygeine und ihre Grenzgebiete* (Race hygiene and its fringes). Leipzig: Georg Thime Verlag.

Ritter, R. (1940–1941). Die Bestandaufnahme der Zigeuner und Zigeunermischlinge in

Deutschland (Taking inventory of Gypsies and Gypsy breeds). In *Der Öffentliche Gesundheitsdienst* 6B (p. 481). Leipzig: Georg Thime Verlag.

Rose, R., & Weiss, W. (1991). *Sinti und Roma im Dritten Reich: Das Programm der Vernichtung durch Arbeit* (Sinti and Roma in the Third Reich: The program for annihilation by work). Göttingen: Lamur Verlag.

Rosenthal, G. (1997). *Der Holocaust im Leben von drei Generationen: Familien von Überlebenden der Shoah und von Nazi-Tätern* (The Holocaust in the life of three generations: Families of survivors of Shoah and Nazi perpetrators). Gießen: Psychosozial-Verlag.

Roth, S. (1993). The shadow of the Holocaust. In R. Moses (Ed.), *Persistent shadows of the Holocaust: The meaning to those not directly affected* (pp. 37–79). Madison, CT: International Universities Press.

Sandler, J. (1960). The background of safety. *International Journal of Psycho-Analysis, 41,* 352–356.

Scheffel-Baars, G. (1998). My contra-program: A response to my father. In J. S. Kestenberg & C. Kahn (Eds.), *Children surviving persecution: An international study of trauma and healing.* Westport, CT: Praeger Press.

Schneider, C. (1993). Jenseits der Schuld? Die Unfähigkeit zu trauern in der zweiten Generation (Beyond guilt? The inability to mourn in the second generation). *Psyche, 47,* 754–774.

Schur, M. (1955). Comments on the metapsychology of somatization. *The Psychoanalytic Study of the Child, 10,* 119–164. New York: International Universities Press.

Searles, H. F. (1959). The effort to drive the other person crazy: An element in the aetiology and psychotherapy of schizophrenia. In *Collected papers on schizophrenia and related subjects* (pp. 254–283). New York: International Universities Press.

Searles, H. F. (1979). *Countertransference and related subjects.* New York: International Universities Press.

Shanfield, S. B., Swain, B. J., & Benjamin, G. A. H. (1986–87). Parents' responses to the death of adult children from accidents and cancer: A comparison. *Omega, 17,* 289–297.

Shengold, L. (1989). *Soul murder: The effect of childhood abuse and deprivation.* New Haven, CT: Yale University Press.

Sievers, B. (1999). *Socio-analysis of war.* Bergische Universität Wuppertal (unpublished monograph).

Siewert, K. (Ed.). (1996). *Rotwelsch-Dialekte: Symposion Münster 10. bis 12. März 1995* (Rotwelsh dialects: Symposium in Münster, March 10–12, 1995). Wiesbaden: Harrassowitz Verlag.

Solnit, A. J. (1987). A psychoanalytic view of play. *Psychoanalytic Study of the Child, 42,* 205–219.

Sonnenberg, S. M. (1974). Children of survivors. *Journal of the American Psychoanalytic Association, 22,* 200–204.

Spitz, R. A. (1957). *No and yes: On the beginning of human communication.* New York: International Universities Press.

Spitz, R. A. (1965). *The first year of life: A psychoanalytic study of normal and deviant development of object relations.* New York: International Universities Press.

Stern, D. N. (1985). *The interpersonal world of the infant.* New York: Basic Books.

Stern, J. (2000a). Personal communication with V. D. Volkan.

Stern, J. (2000b). Psychological aspects of the trial of Adolf Eichmann. *Mind and Human Interaction, 11,* 127–144.

Stewart, S. (1956). *Give us this day*. New York: Avon Books (1990).

Streeck-Fischer, A. (1999). Naziskins in Germany: How traumatization deals with the past. *Mind and Human Interaction, 10,* 84–97

Sullivan, H. S. (1962). *Schizophrenia as a human process*. New York: W. W. Norton.

Tähkä, V. (1984). Dealing with object loss. *Scandinavian Psychoanalytic Review, 1,* 13–33.

Tähkä, V. (1988). On the early formation of the mind. II: From differentiation to self and object constancy. *Psychoanalytic Study of the Child 43,* 101–134. New Haven, CT: Yale University Press.

Tähkä, V. (1993). *Mind and its treatment: A psychoanalytic approach*. Madison, CT: International Universities Press.

Terry, D. J. (1984). The damaging effects of the "survivor syndrome." In S. A. Luel & P. Marcus (Eds.), *Psychoanalytic reflections on the Holocaust: Selected essays* (pp. 134–148). New York: Ktav.

Thomson, J. A. (2000). Terror, tears, and timelessness: Individual and group responses to trauma. *Mind and Human Interaction, 11,* 162–176.

Volkan, V. D. (1976). *Primitive internalized object relations: A clinical study of schizophrenic, borderline, and narcissistic patients*. New York: International Universities Press.

Volkan, V. D. (1979). *Cyprus: War and adaptation*. Charlottesville, VA: The University Press of Virginia.

Volkan, V. D. (1981). *Linking objects and linking phenomena: A study of forms, symptoms, metapsychology and therapy of complicated mourning*. New York: International Universities Press.

Volkan, V. D. (1987). *Six steps in the treatment of borderline personality organization*. Northvale, NJ: Jason Aronson.

Volkan, V. D. (1988). *The need to have enemies and allies: From clinical practice to international relationships*. Northvale, NJ: Jason Aronson.

Volkan, V. D. (1991a). On chosen trauma. *Mind and Human Interaction, 4,* 3–19.

Volkan, V. D. (1991b). The intrapsychic story of integration in a borderline patient. In L. B. Boyer & P. L. Giovacchini (Eds.), *Master clinicians on treating the regressed patient*, Vol. 2 (pp. 279–297). Northvale, NJ: Jason Aronson.

Volkan, V. D. (1992). Ethnonationalistic rituals: An introduction. *Mind and Human Interaction, 4,* 3–19.

Volkan, V. D. (1993). Immigrants and refugees: A psychodynamic perspective. *Mind and Human Interaction, 4,* 63–69.

Volkan, V. D. (1995). *The infantile psychotic self and its fates: Understanding and treating schizophrenics and other difficult patients*. Northvale, NJ: Jason Aronson.

Volkan, V. D. (1997a). The seed of madness. In V. D. Volkan & S. Akhtar (Eds.), *The seed of madness: Constitution, environment, and fantasy in the organization of the psychotic core* (pp. 3–16). Madison, CT: International Universities Press.

Volkan, V. D. (1997b). *Bloodlines: From ethnic pride to ethnic terrorism*. New York: Farrar, Straus, & Giroux.

Volkan, V. D. (1999a). *Das Versagen der Diplomatie: Zur Psychoanalyse nationaler, ethnischer und religiöser Konflikte* (The failure of diplomacy: The psychoanalysis of national, ethnic and religious conflicts). Gießen: Psychosozial-Verlag.

Volkan, V. D. (1999b). Psychoanalysis and diplomacy, Part 1: Individual and large-group identity. *Journal of Applied Psychoanalytic Studies, 1,* 29–55.

Volkan, V. D. (1999c). Psychoanalysis and diplomacy, Part 2: Large-group rituals. *Journal of Applied Psychoanalytic Studies, 1,* 223–247.

Volkan, V. D. (1999d). Childhood sibling rivalry and unconscious womb fantasies in adults. In S. Akhtar & S. Kramer (Eds.), *Brothers and sisters: Developmental, dynamic, and technical aspects of the sibling relationship* (pp. 113–134). Northvale, NJ: Jason Aronson.

Volkan, V. D. (1999e). Post-traumatic states: Beyond individual PTSD in societies ravaged by ethnic conflict. *Canadian Foreign Policy, 7,* 27–38.

Volkan, V.D. (2000). Traumatized societies and psychological care: Expanding the concept of preventive medicine. *Mind and Human Interaction, 11,* 177–194.

Volkan, V. D., Akhtar, S., Dorn, R. M., Kafka, J. S., Kernberg, O. F., Olsson, P. A., Rogers, R. R., & Shanfield, S. (1998). Leaders and decision-making. *Mind and Human Interaction, 9,* 130–181.

Volkan, V. D., & Ast, G. (1992). *Eine Borderline-Therapie: Strukturelle und Objektbeziehungskonflikte in der Psychoanalyse der Borderline-Persönlichkeitsorganisation* (On borderline therapy: Structural and object relations conflicts in the psychoanalysis of borderline personality organization). Göttingen: Vandenhoeck & Ruprecht.

Volkan, V. D., & Ast, G. (1994). *Spektrum des Narzißmus: Eine klinische Studie des gesunden Narzißmus, des narzißtisch-masochistischen Charakters, der narzißtischen Persönlichkeitsorganisation, des malignen Narzißmus und des erfolgreichen Narzißmus* (On the spectrum of narcissism: A clinical study of healthy narcissism, narcissistic-masochistic character, narcissistic personality organization, malignant narcissism and successful narcissism). Göttingen, Germany: Vandenhoeck & Ruprecht.

Volkan, V. D., & Ast, G. (1997). *Siblings in the unconscious and psychopathology.* Madison, CT: International Universities Press.

Volkan, V. D., & Ast, G. (in press). Curing Gitta's "leaking body": Actualized unconscious fantasies and therapeutic play. *Journal of Clinical Psychoanalysis.*

Volkan, V. D., & Berent, S. (1976). Psychiatric aspects of surgical treatment for problems of sexual identification (transsexualism). In J. G. Howells (Ed.), *Modern perspectives in the psychiatric aspects of surgery* (pp. 447–467). New York: Brunner/Mazel.

Volkan, V. D., & Greer, W. F. (1995). True transsexualism. In I. Rosen (Ed.), *Sexual deviations* (pp. 158–173). London: Oxford University Press.

Volkan, V. D., & Itzkowitz, N. (1994). *Turks and Greeks: Neighbors in conflict.* Cambridgeshire, England: Eothen Press.

Volkan, V. D., & Masri, A. (1989). The development of female transsexualism. *American Journal of Psychotherapy, 43,* 92–107.

Volkan, V. D., & Zintl, E. (1993). *Life after loss: The lessons of grief.* New York: Charles Scribner's Sons.

Wardi, D. (1992). *Memorial candles: Children of the Holocaust.* London: Tavistock.

Werman, D. S. (1984). The premature transference. Paper presented at the American Psychoanalytic Association Meeting, San Diego, California, May 16–20.

Werner, H., & Kaplan, B. (1963). *Symbol formation.* New York: Wiley.

Williams, R. M., & Parkes, C. M. (1975). Psychosocial effects of disaster: Birth rate in Aberfan. *British Medical Journal, 2,* 303–304.

Winnicott, D. W. (1953). Transitional objects and transitional phenomena. *International Journal of Psycho-Analysis, 34,* 89–97.

Winnicott, D. W. (1960). The theory of the parent–infant relationship. In *Maturational processes and the facilitating environment* (pp. 37–45). New York: International Universities Press, 1965.

Winnik, H. Z. (1968). Contribution to symposium on psychic traumatization through social catastrophe. *International Journal of Psycho-Analysis, 49,* 298–305.

Wolf, S. A. (1956). *Wörterbuch des Rotwelschen: Deutsche Gaunersprache* (Dictionary of Rotwelsch: German language of petty criminals). Mannheim: Bibliographisches Institut.

Wolfenstein, M. (1966). How is mourning possible? *The Psychoanalytic Study of the Child, 21,* 93–123. New York: International Universities Press.

Wolfenstein, M. (1969). Loss, rage, and repetition. *The Psychoanalytic Study of the Child, 24,* 432–460. New York: International Universities Press.

World Health Organization and United Nations High Commissioner for Refugees (1996). *Mental health of refugees.* Geneva: World Health Organization.

Yablonka, H. (1994). *Foreign brethren: Holocaust survivors in the State of Israel 1948–1952.* Beersheva, Israel: Yad Izhak Ben Zwi Press and Ben Gurion University Press. (In Hebrew.)

Yaşın, Ö. (1965). *Oğlum Savaş'a Mektuplar* (Letters to my son Savaş). Nicosia, Cyprus: Çevre Yayınları.

Zuckerman, R., & Volkan, V. D. (1988). Complicated mourning over a body defect: The making of a "living linking object." In D. Deitrich & P. Shabad (Eds.), *The problem of loss and mourning: Psychoanalytic perspectives* (pp. 257–274). New York: International Universities Press.

Index